COSMOPOLITAN
SHORT CUTS TO
LOOKING GOOD
& FEELING GREAT

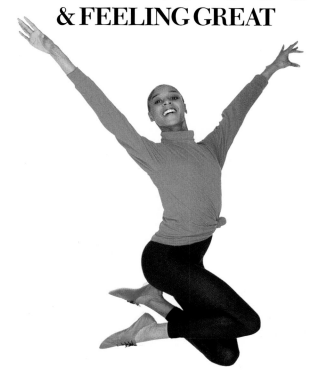

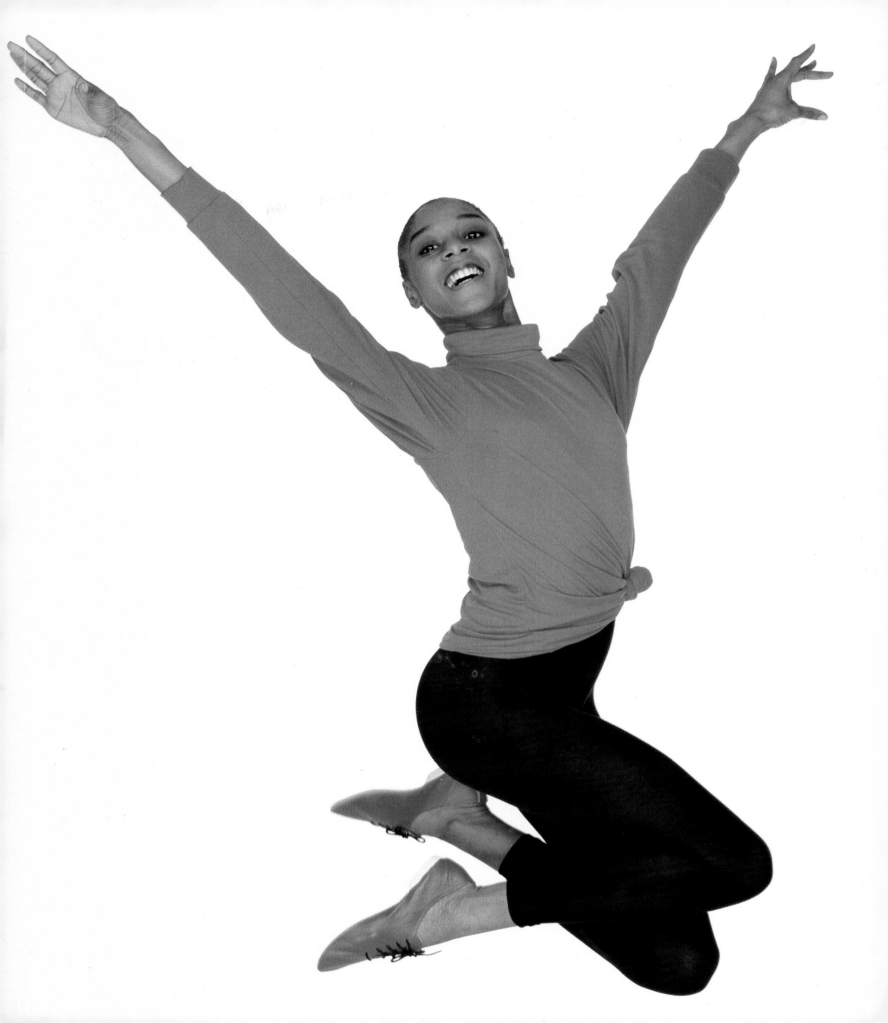

COSMOPOLITAN
SHORT CUTS TO
LOOKING GOOD
& FEELING GREAT

Eileen Mclean:
H, Regent Court
Quarry Corner
Dundonald

CHRISSIE PAINELL & EVE CAMERON

Conran Octopus

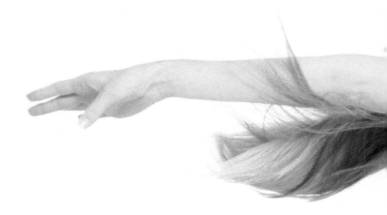

For Brenda and Jill
and Renate and Gilly

First published in 1989 by
Conran Octopus Limited
37 Shelton Street
London WC2H 9HN

ISBN 1 85029 281 7

Project Editor Cortina Butler
Art Editor Karen Bowen
Picture Research Jessica Walton, Joan Tinney
Production Michel Blake
Copy Editor Michelle Clark
Editorial Assistant Rosanna Kelly
Photographers Anthony Crickmay, Iain Philpott
Illustrators Lynne Robinson, Barbara Mullarney Wright

Printed in Hong Kong

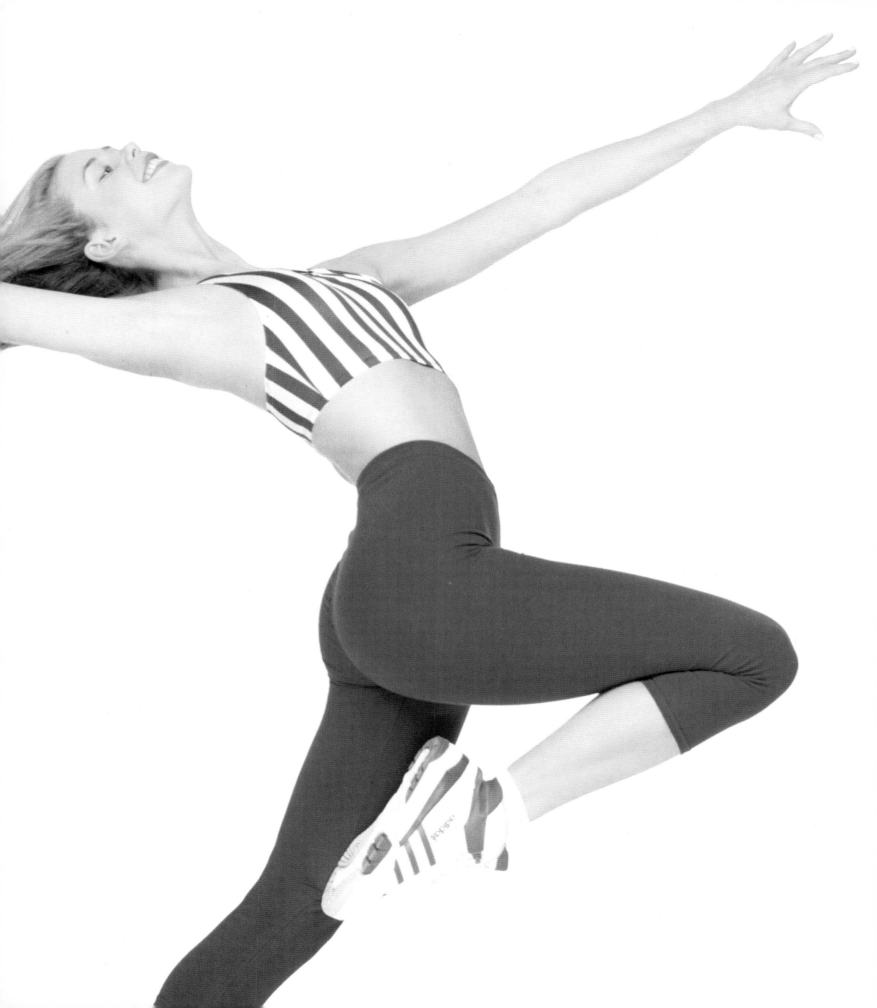

CONTENTS

HAIRCARE 96

THE BODY BEAUTIFUL 120

CLOTHES CONFIDENCE 144

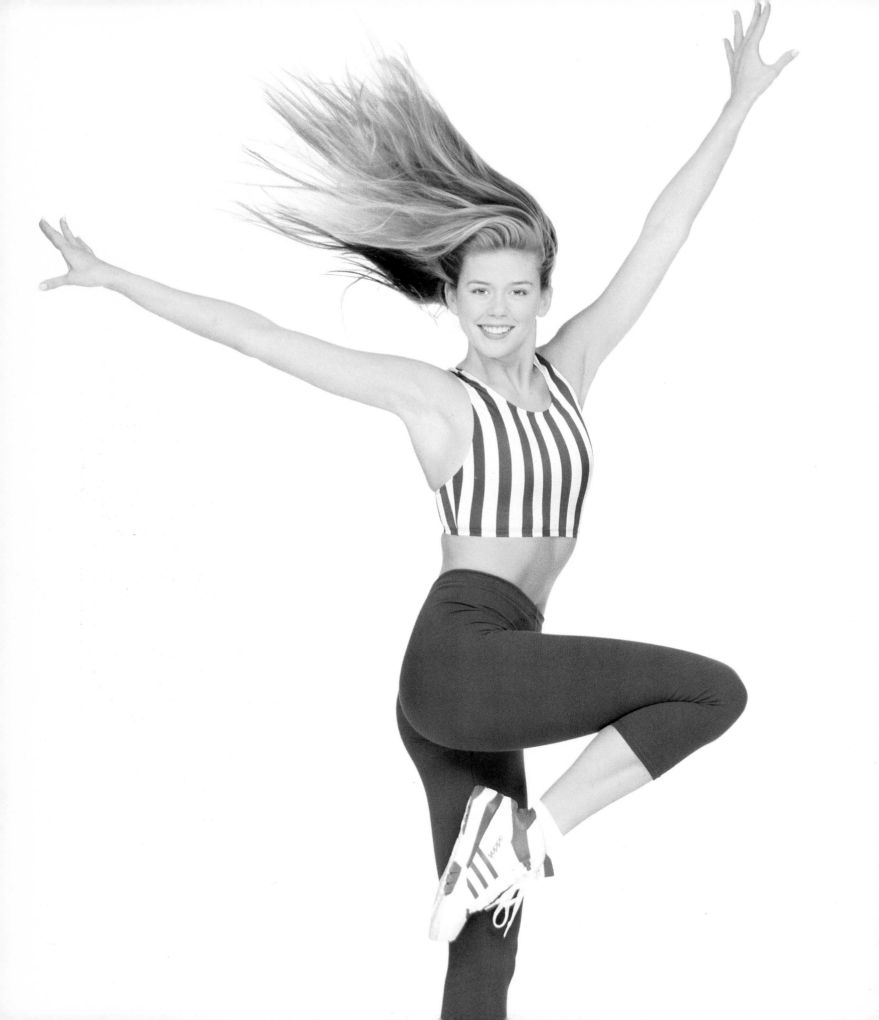

INTRODUCTION

Why not be oneself? That is the whole secret of a successful appearance.

Edith Sitwell

Beauty today no longer means conforming to ideals. Although we all care about our appearance, we are allowed to be very different: modern women come in all shapes and sizes, can be blonde, brunette or redheaded and have widely varying features. In fact, the contemporary approach to beauty positively encourages an emphasis on individuality.

Perhaps the most important change in our concept of beauty in recent years is the shift of focus from accepted standards of appearance to vitality and confidence. These ageless qualities are surely the greatest beauty secrets of all! Taking care of your well-being on a daily basis not only makes you feel more energetic, but will also be reflected in glossy hair, good skin and a fit body.

Nowadays make-up should be used to enhance, rather than disguise, our facial features. It should be light and natural-looking, not a heavy mask. Clothes, too, are more of a personal statement. We no longer have to conform to the dictates of fashion, but instead choose clothes that suit our life-style and personality.

As the pace of our lives accelerates, it has become essential that beauty and fitness should be fitted-into our schedules in the shortest time possible. And, after all, who would want them to be a full-time occupation?

As health and beauty editors of *Cosmopolitan* magazine, we believe strongly that beauty, health and vitality-boosting programmes should take the short cut route – that wherever possible they should be fast, and also fun, to do. We know that once you have mastered the basics and have the quick-fix tricks at your fingertips, you will be equipped to make the most of your looks in minutes, not hours!

So in this book we have cut lengthy routines. We have tailored the key beauty systems to your skin type and to the environment that you live in. We have quizzed make-up artists for the fastest make-up hints and gathered all the hair care wisdom and styling inspiration you will ever need.

Try the fitness workouts that have been designed to firm your body faster than you thought possible! And read the chapter on clothes confidence and personal style that will show you how to create fabulous looks from your wardrobe.

In addition to terrific time-savers and style suggestions, we have put together hundreds of health tips to ensure that you feel your best every day. We hope you enjoy *Short Cuts to Looking Good and Feeling Great*. You will soon wonder how you managed without it!

Chrissie Painell

Eve Cameron

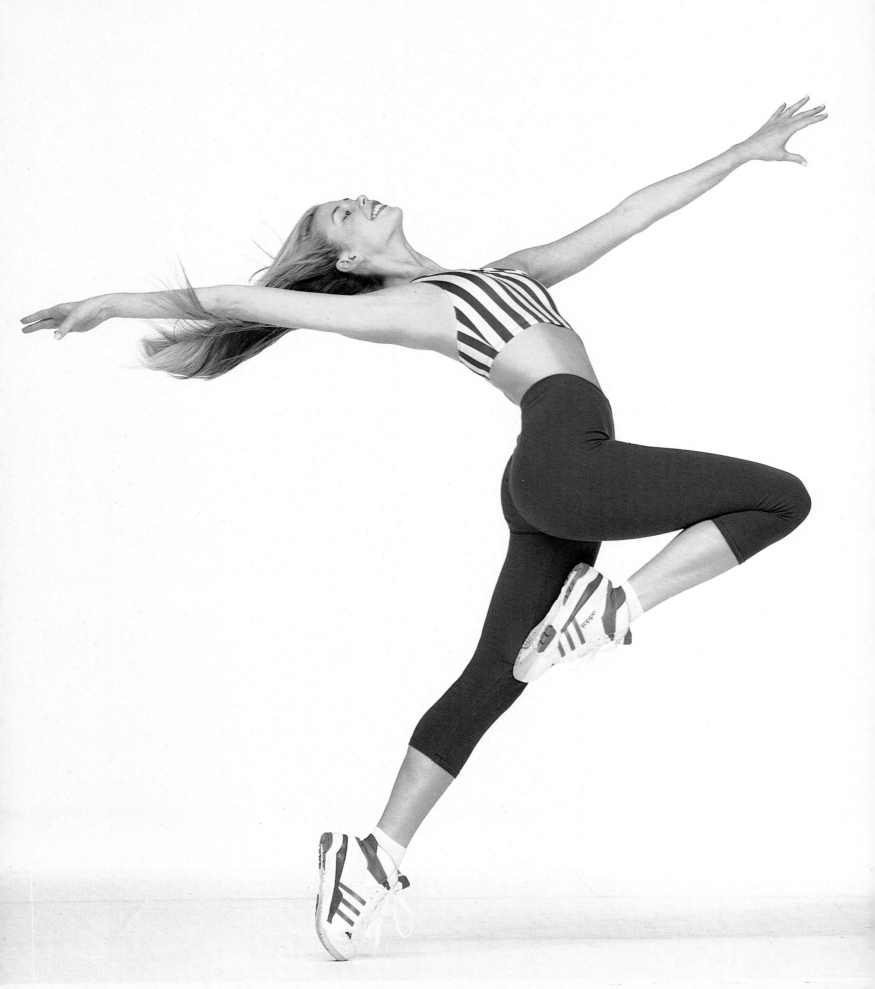

WELL-BEING

What are the vital elements that keep your well-being high?
First a varied and nutritious diet. Next, regular exercise
to increase energy levels and build a stronger body.
And last, but definitely not least, stress-beating strategies
to help you relax and enjoy life. Use our health secrets
and you'll feel better than ever in just a few days!

HEALTHY EATING

Natural, nutritious food is a vital ingredient in a healthy life-style.
Here are easy ways to develop good food habits.

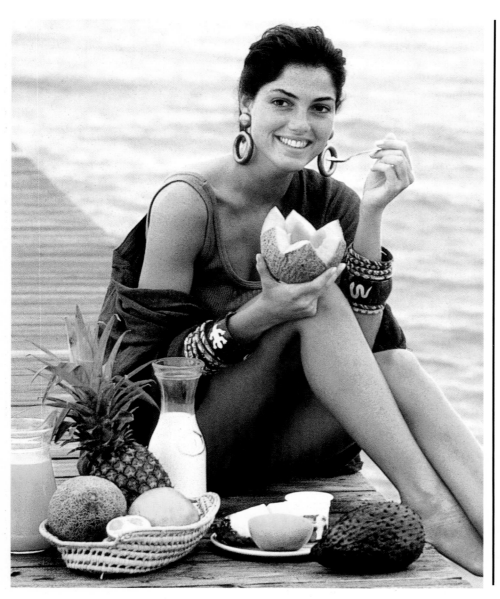

Would you like to switch to a healthier diet but find that you just can't resist the daily chocolate bar and non-stop cups of coffee? Are you too tired after a long day to make a salad and find that you open a pre-packed meal instead?

Of course none of these eating habits will harm you, provided that they are not the staples of your daily diet. The foundation of healthy eating is ensuring that you supply your body with all the nutritious items it needs and cut down on the extras that are not so good for you.

EATING FOR ENERGY AND HEALTH

These food tips form the building blocks of an energizing diet.

Eat fresh fruit, vegetables and salads daily

These are all storehouses of vitamins and minerals that also supply vital fibre. Eat a small salad at lunch-time and fresh vegetables with your evening meal, plus fruit for dessert. For a sweet but healthy treat, look out for exotic fruits such as mango or papaya.

Eat fish twice a week

Oily fish contains Omega–3 oil, which helps protect us from heart disease. Build up a repertoire of healthy meals that are fast to make.

Make sure that the meat content of your meal is the smallest proportion
Aim for a meat content of about 20 per cent, with grains and vegetables making up the rest of the main course. Limit your intake of red meat to twice a week and always choose lean meat. Chicken, turkey and rabbit are low-fat choices. Always remove the skin of poultry, as it is very fatty. Beef is a better choice than lamb or pork, provided it is lean.

Buy skimmed milk and low-fat yogurts
Adding non-fat dried milk powder to skimmed milk will make it thicker if you find skimmed milk too thin for your taste.

Choose sorbets for desserts instead of ice-cream
Use low-fat yogurt or fromage frais instead of full cream, too – they're delicious alternatives.

Eat your main meal before 3 pm
Our metabolism peaks at 12 noon so nutritionists advise that we eat the majority of our food by 3 pm, particularly protein and fatty foods.

ENERGY BREAKFAST
Kick off your day with a glass of hot water and lemon, adding a small amount of clear honey if you wish. It's refreshing and cleansing to your system.

Make your breakfast a combination of protein and complex carbohydrates. Cereals are a good source of fibre. Top them with seeds, such as delicious pumpkin seeds, and chopped nuts. Soak sugar-free muesli and some dried fruit in a little apple juice overnight for added sweetness. Low-fat yogurt provides protein and calcium. Toast provides fibre and carbohydrates. Try it with sugar-free fruit spread (but not butter).

FAST MEAL TIPS
Healthy food does not have to be time-consuming to prepare – there are plenty of fast food options that also do you good.
● Steaming vegetables is just as fast as boiling and preserves more nutrients. They should be cooked to the point where they are tender but still crisp.
● Always keep frozen vegetables in the house. Many of them are just as nutritious as the fresh varieties.
● Eat 50 per cent of your vegetables raw. Serve some as crudités while the food is cooking.
● Quick-cook rice is slightly more processed than plain rice, but is much better for you than a pan of fried potatoes!

● Brown noodles are super-quick to cook and make a delicious base for many dishes.
● Fresh wholewheat spaghetti takes a minute to cook. Serve it with pesto and steamed courgettes.

EASY WAYS TO INCREASE FIBRE INTAKE
Since the beginning of the century, the amount of fibre in the Western diet has dropped by a staggering 75 per cent. At the same time, the incidence of constipation and bowel diseases has risen substantially.

We should be eating approximately 30 g (1 oz) of fibre per day for general health and to avoid diseases of the bowel. Here are some suggestions to help you increase the fibre in your diet.
New forms of fibre These are being introduced into the shops. Mixtures of soluble and insoluble fibre, they are very finely ground and can be mixed instantly into cereals, soups and casseroles.
Bread A slice of wholegrain bread provides 3 g of fibre.
Muesli 1 serving (3 tablespoons) of muesli provides 3 g of fibre.
Fruit Oranges contain 3 g; a pear with skin 3.4 g; apples 2 g.
Vegetables Broccoli contains 1.8 g per spear; spinach 6.3 g per tablespoon; ½ aubergine with the skin left on 3.2 g.

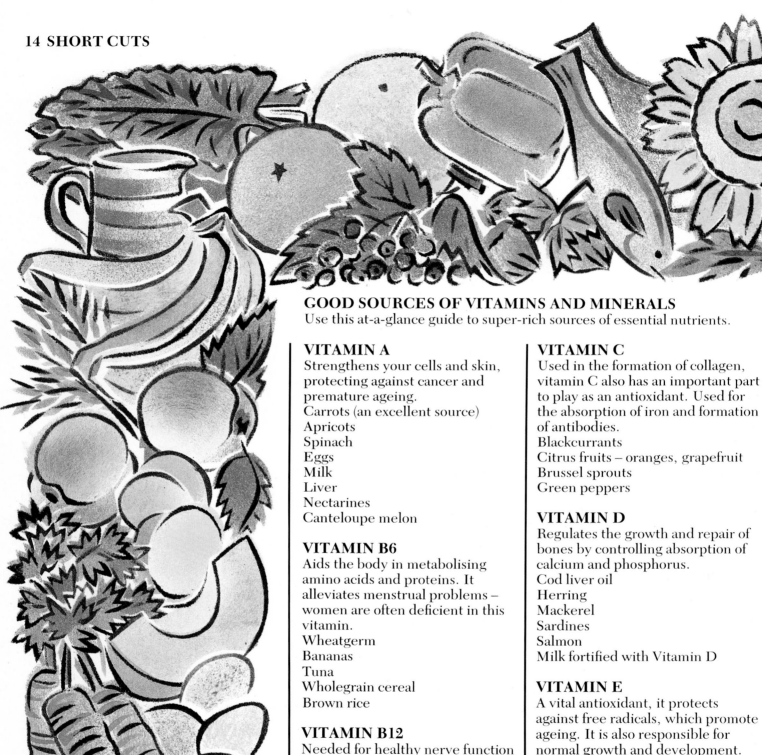

GOOD SOURCES OF VITAMINS AND MINERALS

Use this at-a-glance guide to super-rich sources of essential nutrients.

VITAMIN A
Strengthens your cells and skin, protecting against cancer and premature ageing.
Carrots (an excellent source)
Apricots
Spinach
Eggs
Milk
Liver
Nectarines
Canteloupe melon

VITAMIN B6
Aids the body in metabolising amino acids and proteins. It alleviates menstrual problems – women are often deficient in this vitamin.
Wheatgerm
Bananas
Tuna
Wholegrain cereal
Brown rice

VITAMIN B12
Needed for healthy nerve function and production of red blood cells.
Meat
Eggs
Milk
(Vegetarians are advised to take supplements.)

VITAMIN C
Used in the formation of collagen, vitamin C also has an important part to play as an antioxidant. Used for the absorption of iron and formation of antibodies.
Blackcurrants
Citrus fruits – oranges, grapefruit
Brussel sprouts
Green peppers

VITAMIN D
Regulates the growth and repair of bones by controlling absorption of calcium and phosphorus.
Cod liver oil
Herring
Mackerel
Sardines
Salmon
Milk fortified with Vitamin D

VITAMIN E
A vital antioxidant, it protects against free radicals, which promote ageing. It is also responsible for normal growth and development.
Seeds, such as safflower and sunflower
Nuts, such as almonds, hazelnuts, walnuts
Milk
Wheatgerm
Vegetable oils, such as corn oil

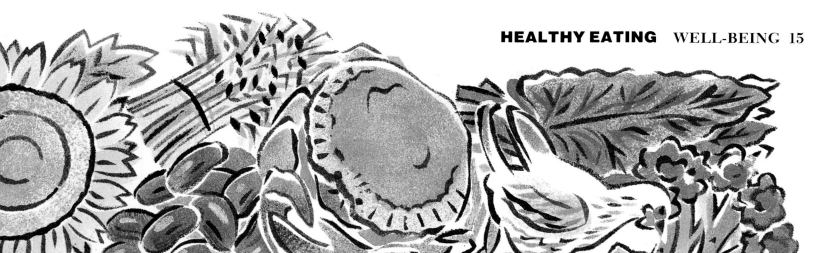

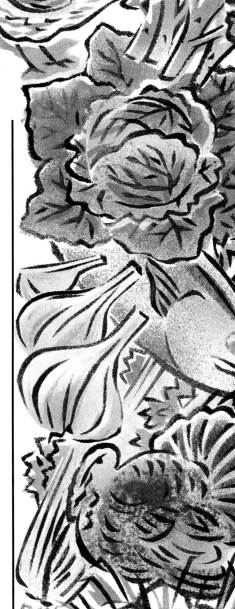

CALCIUM
Helps prevent osteoporosis (brittleness of the bones) which affects many women after the menopause. Builds bones and teeth and helps regulate heartbeat and blood clotting.
Milk
Yogurt
Nuts
Seeds
Broccoli
Green vegetables
Pulses
Fish, particularly sardines, pilchards, whitebait, crab, cod
Rhubarb

IRON
Prevents anaemia, stimulates the production of haemoglobin, which carries oxygen to the cells.
Kidneys
Cane molasses
Tuna fish
Pulses, such as lentils
Seaweed
Wholegrain products
Egg yolk

MAGNESIUM
Aids bone growth and nerve and muscle function.
Cod

Mackerel
Leafy green vegetables
Sunflower seeds

SELENIUM
Complements vitamin E as an antioxidant and promotes growth and development.
Seafood
Tuna
Wheatgerm
Milk
Liver
Chicken
Broccoli
Cabbage
Celery
Garlic

ZINC
Aids wound-healing and promotes cell growth and repair.
Sesame and sunflower seeds
Fish
Milk
Oysters
Pilchards
Wholegrain products
Turkey
Soya beans
Egg yolk

CONTROLLING YOUR WEIGHT

Forget faddy diets. Instead switch to a balanced eating plan to maintain your ideal weight.

It is an established fact that the great majority of diets claiming to make you lose weight *don't work*. When you diet, your body automatically adjusts to the reduction in calories, slowing down the metabolism and therefore burning calories less efficiently. When you resume your usual eating patterns, the weight goes right back on. In addition, when you deprive your body of food, it prefers to derive the energy it needs from your *muscle* instead of using up fat stores, so the weight reduction you see on the scales is actually loss of lean muscle and not just fat.

The good news is that there is an answer. Forget fad diets and don't use very low calorie diets. All of these deplete your energy levels and may even be harmful to your health. Instead you should switch to a *long-term*, sensible, balanced eating plan that is low in fats and sugar. Research at American universities has shown that women who were put on a low-fat diet lost weight even though other foods were not restricted.

It is easy to make a low-fat diet a way of life and, as well as helping weight loss, it is the road to a healthy heart.

CUTTING DOWN THE FAT CONTENT IN YOUR DIET

Fat is not all bad for you – it plays an important role in providing vitamins and aiding their absorption, for example. The chief distinction in different types of fat is between saturated and unsaturated fats. Saturated fats are mostly animal products, unsaturated fats usually come from vegetables (though coconut oil is a saturated fat). Saturated fat appears to increase the cholesterol level of the blood, but there is some evidence that unsaturated fats may reduce it. The first aim, therefore in planning a low-fat diet should be to reduce your consumption of saturated fats. The five leading sources of saturated fat in our diets have been found to be:

- hamburgers
- sausages, hot dogs and ham
- whole milk
- cakes and biscuits
- steaks and roast beef

Limit your intake of these and use the following short cuts to help you lose unwanted pounds.

- Skip butter or margarine on bread and in sandwiches.
- Add extra (low-fat) filling to a jacket potato such as reduced-sugar baked beans, sweet corn and peppers and ratatouille, instead of butter or margarine.

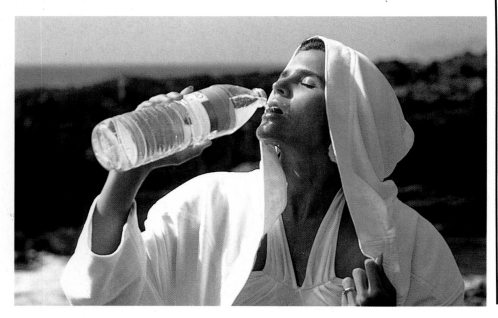

● Squeeze lemon on to salad instead of salad cream or mayonnaise.

● Try to limit the number of ready-prepared dishes you eat – they are often a source of hidden fat, or look for low-fat meals.

● Look closely at food labels – products made with vegetable oils are healthier (unless they contain coconut oil or palm oil, which are very high in saturated fat) but *hydrogenated* vegetable oils are not. These oils have been hardened and turned into saturated fat. Buy extra-virgin olive oil and cold-pressed vegetable oils, such as safflower and sunflower.

● Non-dairy frozen desserts, such as sorbets, are a better choice than ice-cream.

● Chicken is a good protein-packed food, as its fat is mostly mono-unsaturated, a type of fat that appears to lower blood cholesterol. Remove the fatty skin.

When you are trying to lose weight, do not take appetite suppressants (which are sold at some diet clinics) – they can be addictive.

Aerobic exercise is considered by sports scientists to be the best weight-loss workout, as it burns up calories and fat and builds up muscle (see page 19).

If you are undereating, rather than overeating or eating unhealthily, seek expert advice in order to solve any underlying psychological problems you may be experiencing. Your family doctor will be able to refer you to a specialist.

The important factor for all of us to bear in mind is not to become obsessed with food or our body shape – we are, after all, all different – but to try to follow good, general principles of healthy eating as a way of life.

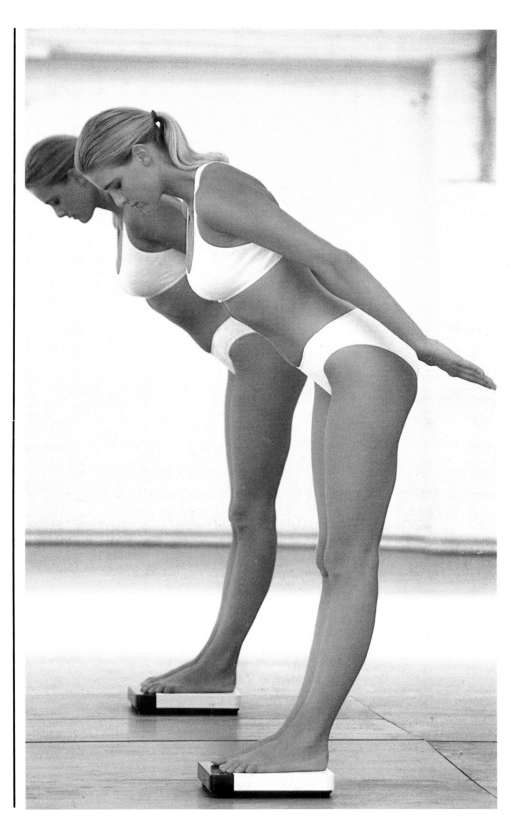

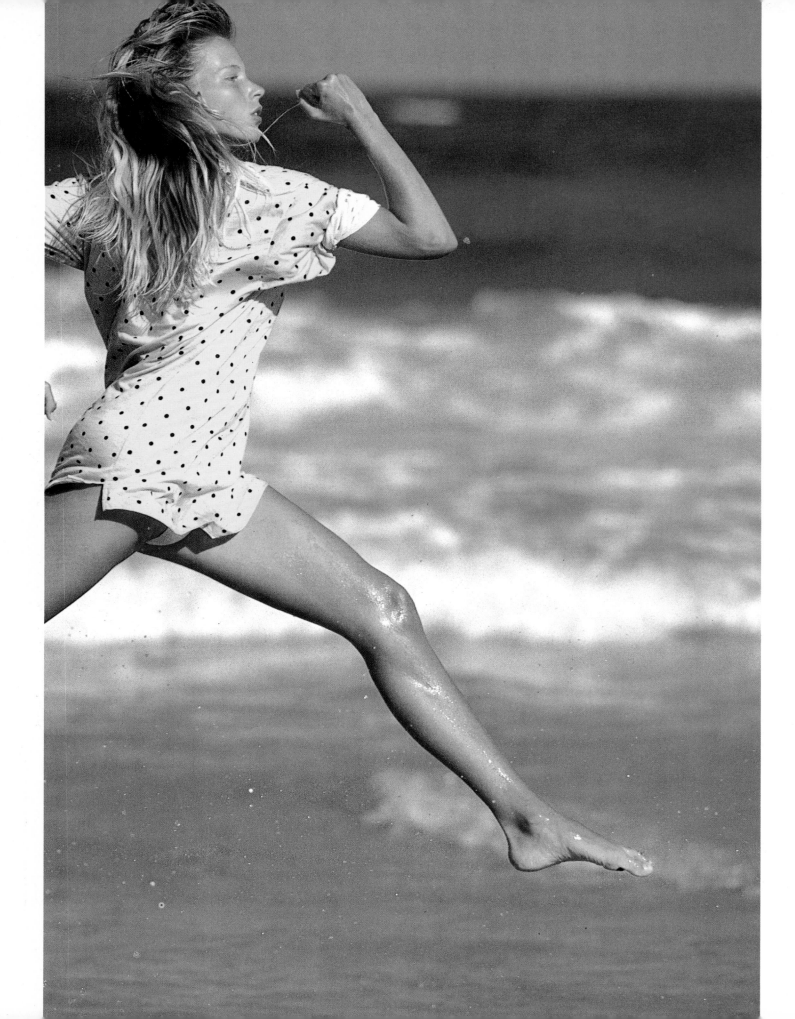

THE VITALITY FACTOR

Exercise gives us the energy to speed through life.
Increase your energy resources today!

Exercising regularly can make a huge difference to your energy levels. Without exercise, we feel sluggish and slow, but when we exercise vigorously the benefits are wide-ranging. Expending energy:
● actually gives you more energy than you had before
● means that nutrients are absorbed more efficiently
● helps to prevent osteoporosis (brittleness of the bones)
● sleeks and shapes your body
● curbs high blood-pressure and dramatically reduces the risk of heart disease
● relaxes you and produces hormones that improve your mood
● burns calories
● improves circulation to the skin
● helps you get a better night's rest.

In order to be fit, we need to ensure that our exercise routine includes all the elements in the exercise equation:
Aerobic exercise to improve our stamina and get our circulation moving faster.
Strengthening exercises to improve muscle tone and power.
Stretching exercises to develop flexibility (it is important that we work to balance strength with stretching ability).
Stress-releasing exercises which often include gentle movements, such as those in yoga that work on energy pathways and on releasing tension in the body (see page 32).

Try to incorporate all these elements into an exercise routine, working out three times a week, exercising aerobically for twenty to thirty minutes in each of these sessions. Unless you are training to compete in a specific sport, this is usually all the exercise you need to keep your heart healthy and maintain general fitness. Rest days are valuable because over-exercising can be counter-productive, leading to over-use injuries, such as the knee problems runners can experience.

AEROBIC EXERCISE

This raises the heart rate, increasing the flow of oxygen to the muscles and organs and, most importantly, to the heart. When exercising aerobically, you should be comfortably out of breath. You can judge this by seeing how well you can keep up a conversation – if you can't talk, you're overdoing it.

There are two main types of aerobic exercise: high-impact and low-impact.

High-impact aerobics involves energetic jumping and bouncing and can put strain on the joints. Low-impact is the new fitness

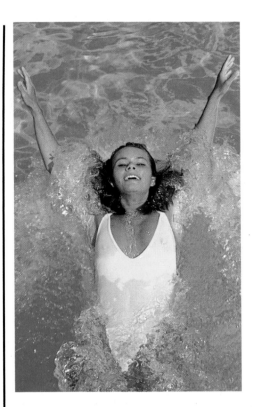

formula that is less stressful. In low-impact aerobic dance classes, you will always have your feet on the floor, cutting out the jogging and the bouncing. The latest thinking is that we don't have to exercise as vigorously as was once believed in order to gain the vitality and health-enhancing results of aerobic activity. Working out at a lower heart rate is just as effective – you just need to exercise longer.

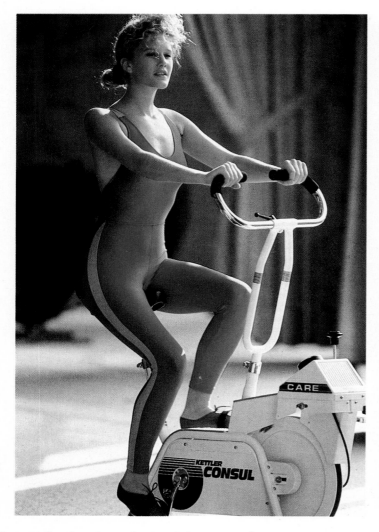
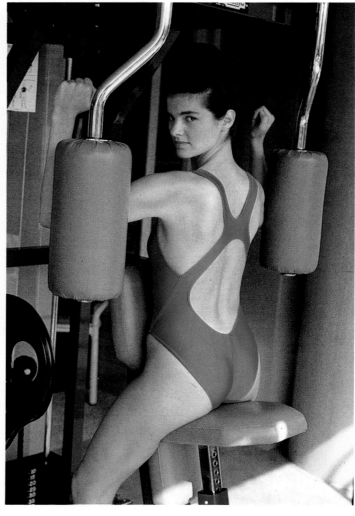

Here's a brief run-down of the different types of aerobic activity you can do:

Cycling or exercise bikes
Very effective forms of low-impact aerobic workout. Strengthens your legs, too.

Rebounding
A rebounder is a mini-trampoline. A fun workout that has the advantage of being low-impact. Rebound aerobic classes are a growing trend in health clubs.

Hydrafitness
A special form of weight-training equipment that is hydraulically driven. The circuit includes rebounders. This is a very - strenuous, low-impact workout, providing strengthening and stamina-improving exercise in super-quick time.

Rowing and rowing machines
This is very effective low-impact exercise, which also builds strength in legs, back and arms.

Swimming
You need to have good technique in order to make this an aerobic workout – a slow breaststroke is unlikely to get your heart rate up, unless you are very unfit. However, if you are a good swimmer, this low-impact activity is an excellent choice of exercise.

Aerobic dance
If you haven't exercised for some time, don't head straight for an aerobics class or buy an aerobics video to use at home. Go to body-conditioning classes first, where you'll be taught body control and good posture. You can then progress to aerobic dance classes and you'll perform the movements safely and effectively. This can be high-impact, low-impact or a combination of both. Before starting

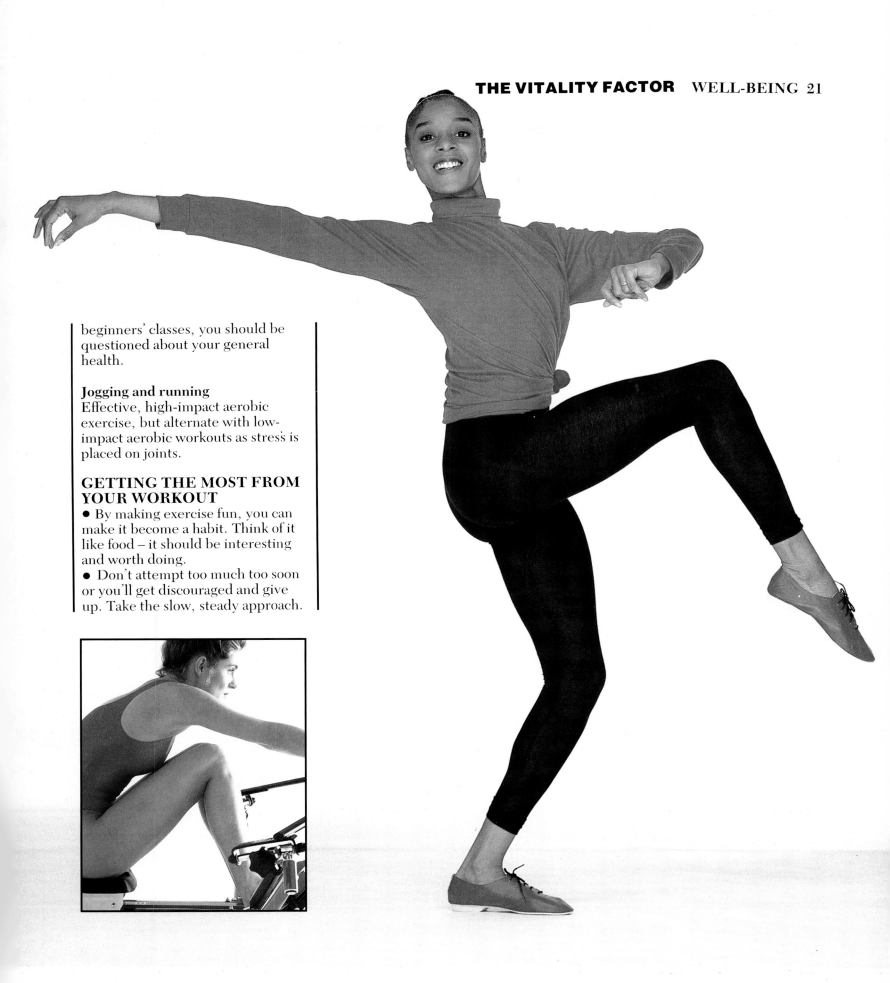

beginners' classes, you should be questioned about your general health.

Jogging and running
Effective, high-impact aerobic exercise, but alternate with low-impact aerobic workouts as stress is placed on joints.

GETTING THE MOST FROM YOUR WORKOUT
● By making exercise fun, you can make it become a habit. Think of it like food – it should be interesting and worth doing.
● Don't attempt too much too soon or you'll get discouraged and give up. Take the slow, steady approach.

SPORTS DIRECTORY

Sporting activities are a fast, fun way to fitness.

Many people prefer to shape up and increase their fitness level through sport instead of doing workout classes. For optimum fitness, the ideal is to incorporate sport into a total fitness programme.

Here you'll find a brief guide to popular sports, their benefits and some easy-to-remember tips. Many provide good aerobic workouts, if played fast enough, and all have body-conditioning advantages. Most importantly, sport is fun, great for de-stressing and a sociable activity offering opportunities to make new friends.

BADMINTON

Badminton is excellent for developing flexibility and eye-hand co-ordination. Strength is not so important for this sport initially, though it will develop as you advance and skills and tricks are usually picked up with practice.

As with tennis and basketball, remember to wear shock-absorbing shoes (for the jumps and lunges).

BASEBALL, SOFTBALL and ROUNDERS

All three are bat and ball games and so throwing and catching are important skills. They help to firm and tone the legs and strengthen the upper body and back. They are not a key means of building

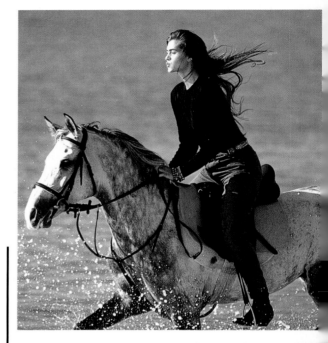

stamina, since running tends to be in short bursts; when your team is batting, quick sprints from base to base are necessary to score runs. You will need to develop flexibility, however, in order to react quickly.

Coaching sessions and team practices usually start with batting, throwing and catching exercises, so you have a chance to improve your technique.

Unless you already have an accurate, long throw, leave deep fielding for a while, as it's easy to overdo it and pull arm muscles.

You'll need to equip yourself with a good pair of running shoes and protective gloves and pads.

BASKETBALL

Basketball is a physically demanding team game, involving quick sprints up and down the court, dribbling and throwing the ball, dodging opponents and shooting to try and score a 'basket'. It provides a good aerobic workout and you will improve co-ordination and flexibility as you practise.

With all the jumping and running, you must wear ankle-supporting, shock-absorbing shoes.

RIDING

Horse-riding does not simply mean sitting there, letting the horse do all the work! You have to give

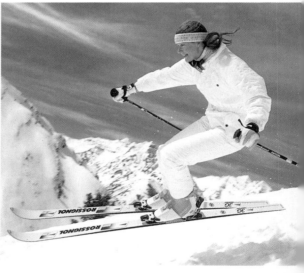

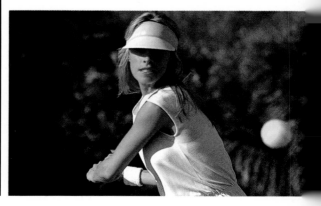

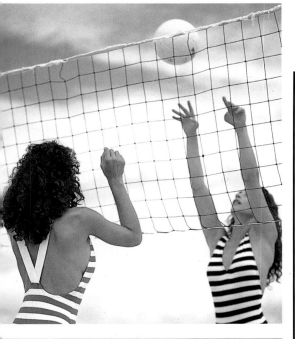

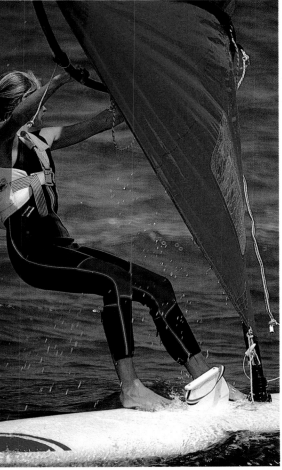

commands, your posture is vital and you need to develop good abdominal control to move with the horse. You will find that it helps to strengthen your back and also strengthens and stretches your thigh and calf muscles.

SAILING

Sailing can be very relaxing, when cruising, for example, or it can be physically challenging, as when yachting in the open seas.

Pulling ropes will strengthen the muscles in your upper back and arms. As you lean out to balance the boat, your abdominal muscles and legs take the strain. Good flexibility is needed to handle a boat when you are changing direction.

SKIING

Skiing is invigorating and exhausting! The fitter you are, though, the less taxing it is. It is necessary to learn correct technique to avoid strains and breaks, and it is wise to do leg-strengthening and stamina building exercises before you head for the slopes. Ski schools will advise on the best exercises to do to prepare yourself.

At beginner's level, you need strength and co-ordination between arms/sticks and legs/skis. As you get more advanced, flexibility becomes increasingly important, particularly if you attempt slalom or jumps.

SURFING

Surfing is a good test of balance and flexibility and builds strength in the lower body. It is wise to learn the basic techniques before setting off to 'catch' your wave.

Being a strong swimmer is essential as you may need to paddle out some distance each time.

TENNIS

With tennis, the level of your game relates directly to its fitness value. A gentle game of doubles is less taxing than a hard-fought singles match, for example.

It is good for developing general fitness and flexibility. You will develop a strong wrist and grip in your racquet arm and footwork is important too. Practise side steps and moving for the ball with backhand and forehand strokes.

Stretch your calf and thigh muscles regularly (see page 136) so that they are less at risk of being pulled.

Before starting a game, warm up your shoulders (see page 122) to reduce the risk of pulled muscles, and wear shock-absorbing shoes.

VOLLEYBALL

Volleyball strengthens the hands and wrists and the pectoral muscles in the chest. You can increase the strength in those areas by hitting the ball with a partner or against the wall. Volleyball also firms and strengthens the legs, particularly the front of the thighs, because of all the jumping, but make sure you've got good shock-absorbing shoes.

WINDSURFING

Windsurfing is good for improving co-ordination and a strong upper body and back is an advantage. It also firms and strengthens your legs.

It is important to have some lessons to learn good techniques in windsurfing or else you will probably never enjoy it. When you have become competent, there are plenty of advanced techniques to learn which will enable you to race and jump waves.

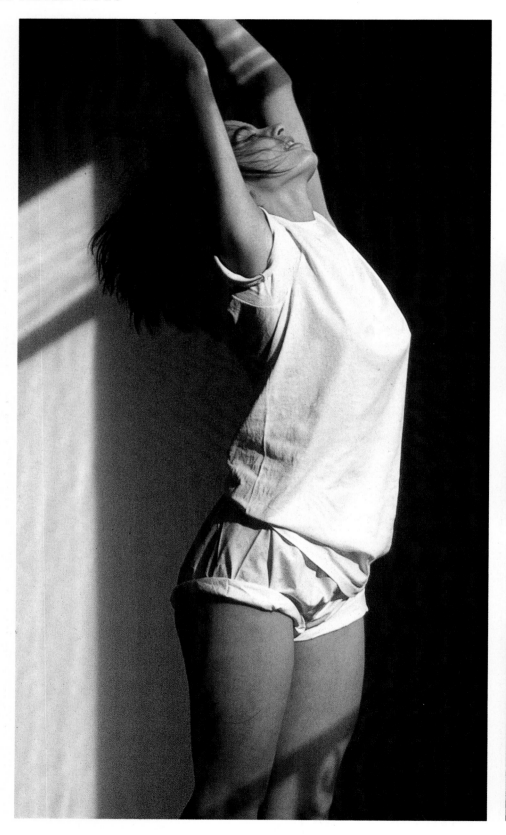

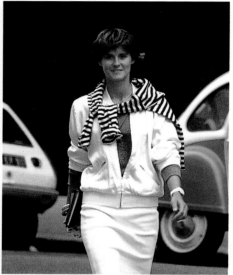

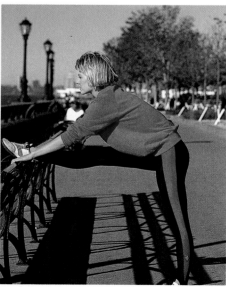

FITTING EXERCISE INTO YOUR DAY

If you are too busy to get to an exercise class, these simple tips will keep you fit while you are on the move.

It can be difficult to schedule exercise sessions when you have a hectic lifestyle. It's a good idea, therefore, to squeeze fitness moves into your day whenever and wherever you have the opportunity! That way you'll maintain your health and increase your energy levels. Here are some ideas.

Try a good morning stretch
It will get the circulation moving on waking up and only takes a few minutes.
● Stand with your feet wide apart and slightly turned out.
● Bend your knees and tuck your buttocks under, pulling your stomach in.
● Now raise your arms slowly and breathe in, stretching up so your legs straighten as you do so.
   Remember to s-t-r-e-t-c-h your arms and whole body up towards the ceiling.
● Lower your arms as you breathe out and bend your knees (check that your knees bend over your feet and do not roll in).
● Breathe in. Repeat the stretch 10 times.

Exercise in the morning
This will ensure that you've slotted it into your day. Get up 20 minutes early a couple of times a week and go for a brisk walk or a gentle jog.

Walk don't ride
Park the car a few streets away or jump off the bus two stops early. Always climb the stairs

Keep moving
If you are sitting at a desk for long periods of time, get up frequently and walk around to keep your circulation moving.

Avoid neck strain
● Tip your chin forwards and swing your head very slowly around to your right.
● Bring your head back to the centre and then sweep around to your left.
● Repeat as often as you wish. *Note*: avoid tipping your head backwards.

Relax your shoulders
Circle your shoulders backwards, lifting them up to your ears and then pulling down so that you can really feel the movement.
   You can also try this shoulder and upper back stretch.
● Bend one arm up behind you and bring your other hand over your shoulder from the front.
● Clasp your hands if you can and gently stretch up. If your hands don't meet, use a scarf to help you.
● Hold for 30 seconds and then swop hands.

Get some fresh air
Go out for a walk *every* lunch-time. A stuffy environment will sap your energy and leave you feeling headachey and lethargic at the end of the day.

Tone your legs and knees
Try the leg-strengthening and knee-toning exercise on page 136.

Keep ankles and wrists supple
Do ankle and wrist circling whenever you remember – while watching television for instance.

Exercise at home
Buy an exercise video to use at home, if you have a video cassette recorder. If you don't have time to do the whole programme, just do the stretching as this is wonderfully relaxing. Warm up for a few minutes first by walking around the room, briskly, circling your arms.

Loosen up your back
Use this lower back stretch whenever the muscles feel tight. It's especially relaxing at the end of a long day.
● Lie on the floor and bend your knees up to your chest.
● Bring your hands round to clasp your legs and rock very gently.
● Relax for a few moments afterwards and then get up slowly.

15-MINUTE SHAPE UP

Our super-effective workout will keep you in fabulous shape.

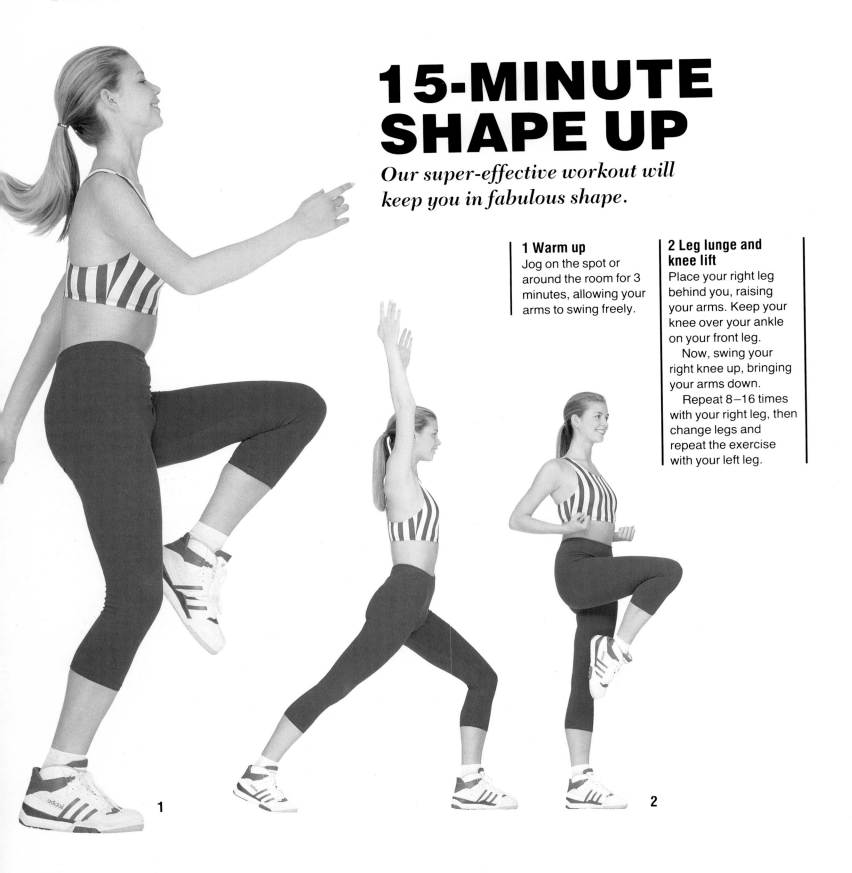

1 Warm up
Jog on the spot or around the room for 3 minutes, allowing your arms to swing freely.

2 Leg lunge and knee lift
Place your right leg behind you, raising your arms. Keep your knee over your ankle on your front leg.

Now, swing your right knee up, bringing your arms down.

Repeat 8–16 times with your right leg, then change legs and repeat the exercise with your left leg.

1

2

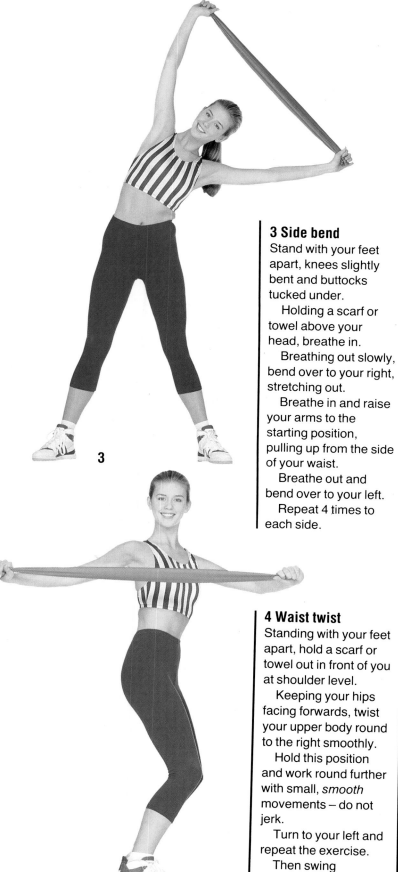

3 Side bend

Stand with your feet apart, knees slightly bent and buttocks tucked under.

Holding a scarf or towel above your head, breathe in.

Breathing out slowly, bend over to your right, stretching out.

Breathe in and raise your arms to the starting position, pulling up from the side of your waist.

Breathe out and bend over to your left.

Repeat 4 times to each side.

4 Waist twist

Standing with your feet apart, hold a scarf or towel out in front of you at shoulder level.

Keeping your hips facing forwards, twist your upper body round to the right smoothly.

Hold this position and work round further with small, *smooth* movements – do not jerk.

Turn to your left and repeat the exercise.

Then swing smoothly from side to side 16 times.

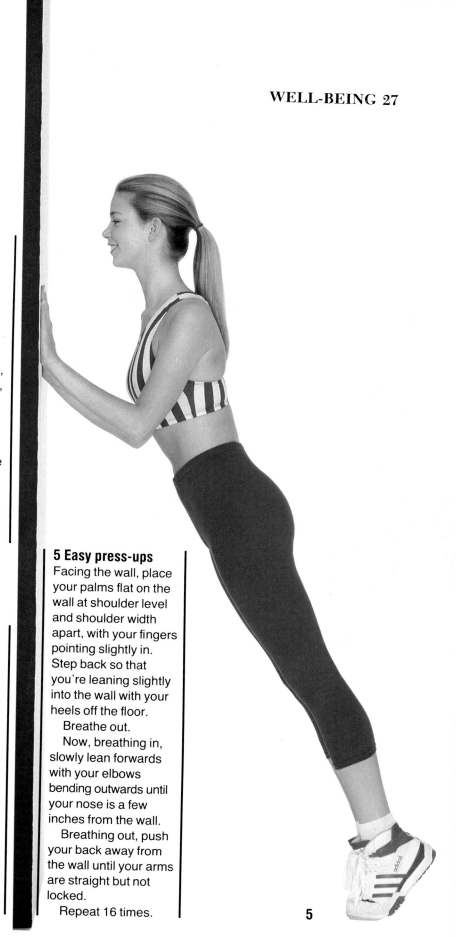

5 Easy press-ups

Facing the wall, place your palms flat on the wall at shoulder level and shoulder width apart, with your fingers pointing slightly in. Step back so that you're leaning slightly into the wall with your heels off the floor.

Breathe out.

Now, breathing in, slowly lean forwards with your elbows bending outwards until your nose is a few inches from the wall.

Breathing out, push your back away from the wall until your arms are straight but not locked.

Repeat 16 times.

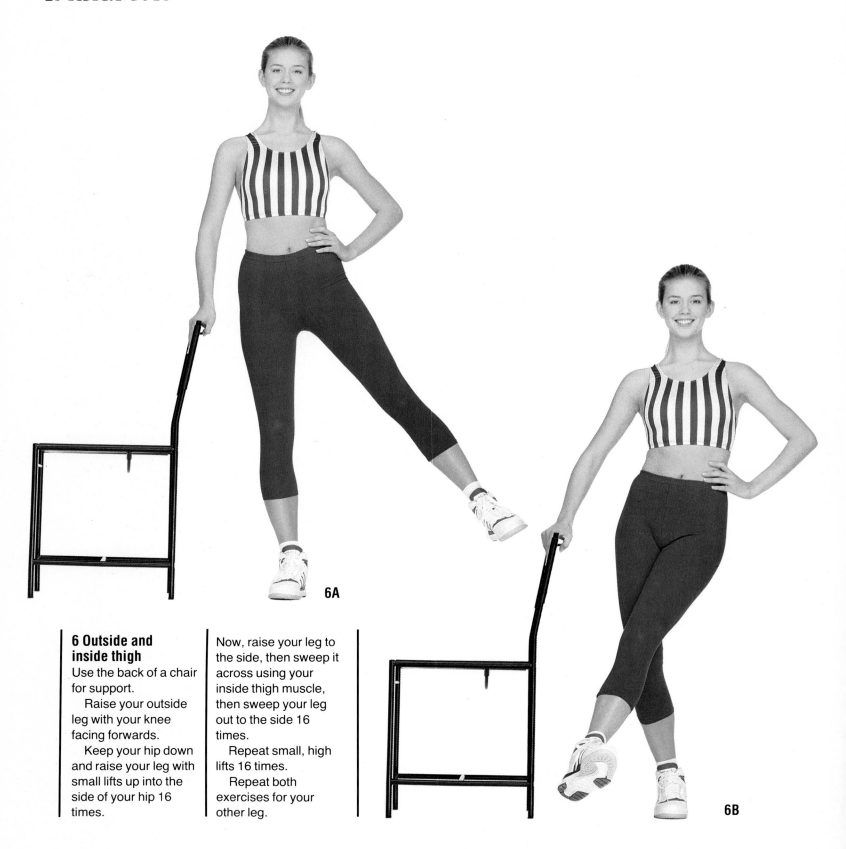

6A

6B

6 Outside and inside thigh

Use the back of a chair for support.

Raise your outside leg with your knee facing forwards.

Keep your hip down and raise your leg with small lifts up into the side of your hip 16 times.

Now, raise your leg to the side, then sweep it across using your inside thigh muscle, then sweep your leg out to the side 16 times.

Repeat small, high lifts 16 times.

Repeat both exercises for your other leg.

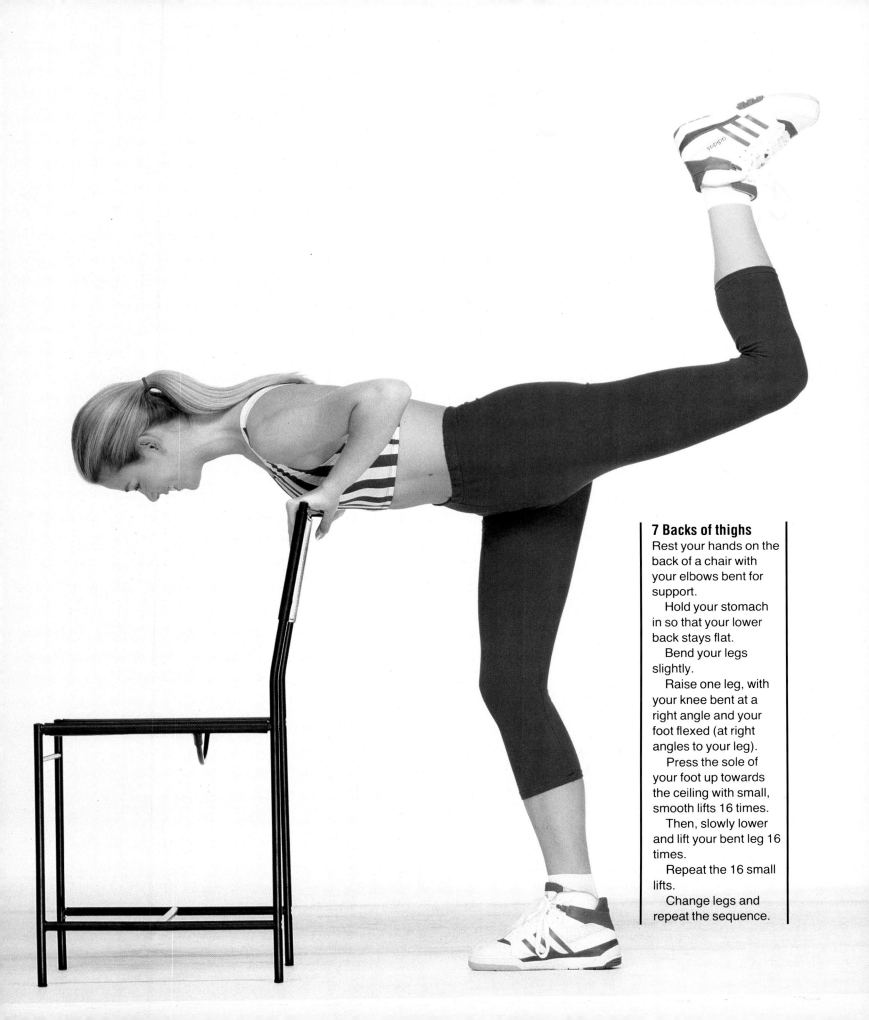

7 Backs of thighs

Rest your hands on the back of a chair with your elbows bent for support.

Hold your stomach in so that your lower back stays flat.

Bend your legs slightly.

Raise one leg, with your knee bent at a right angle and your foot flexed (at right angles to your leg).

Press the sole of your foot up towards the ceiling with small, smooth lifts 16 times.

Then, slowly lower and lift your bent leg 16 times.

Repeat the 16 small lifts.

Change legs and repeat the sequence.

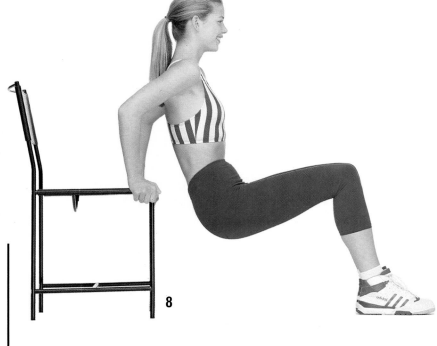

8 Backs of arms
Place your hands on either side of the front of a chair seat, with your back facing the seat.

Place your feet forward so that your bottom drops comfortably and your body-weight is held by your arms.

Bend your elbows, lowering your body, then straighten your arms smoothly, keeping your shoulders down.

Repeat 16 times.
Note: do not try to push up using your thighs or your bottom – only your arms should be working.

9 Stomach
Sit in the middle of a chair with your hands placed on either side of the front of the seat.

Pull your stomach in so that your lower back rounds slightly.

Breathe normally.

Holding your stomach in, draw your right knee up to your chest, then lower it with control. Then draw your left knee up and lower it.

Repeat 8 times with each leg.

To increase the resistance, draw both your knees up to your chest.
Note: make sure that your stomach muscles are taking the weight of your legs – you should not feel *any* pull in your lower back.

Now, lie on the floor with legs bent up at right angles, supported by a chair seat.

Pull your stomach in so that your lower back presses into the floor.

Place your hands lightly under your head with your elbows dropped out to each side.

Raise and lower your head, shoulders and upper back, feeling your abdominal muscles working.

Breathe in, then breathe out as you lift up, breathe in as you lower down with control.

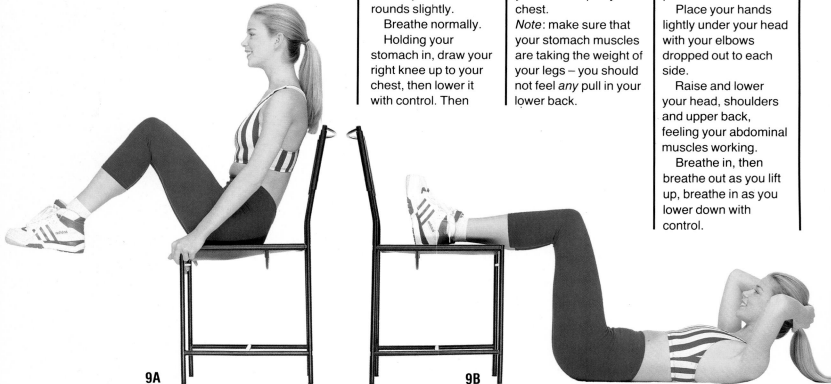

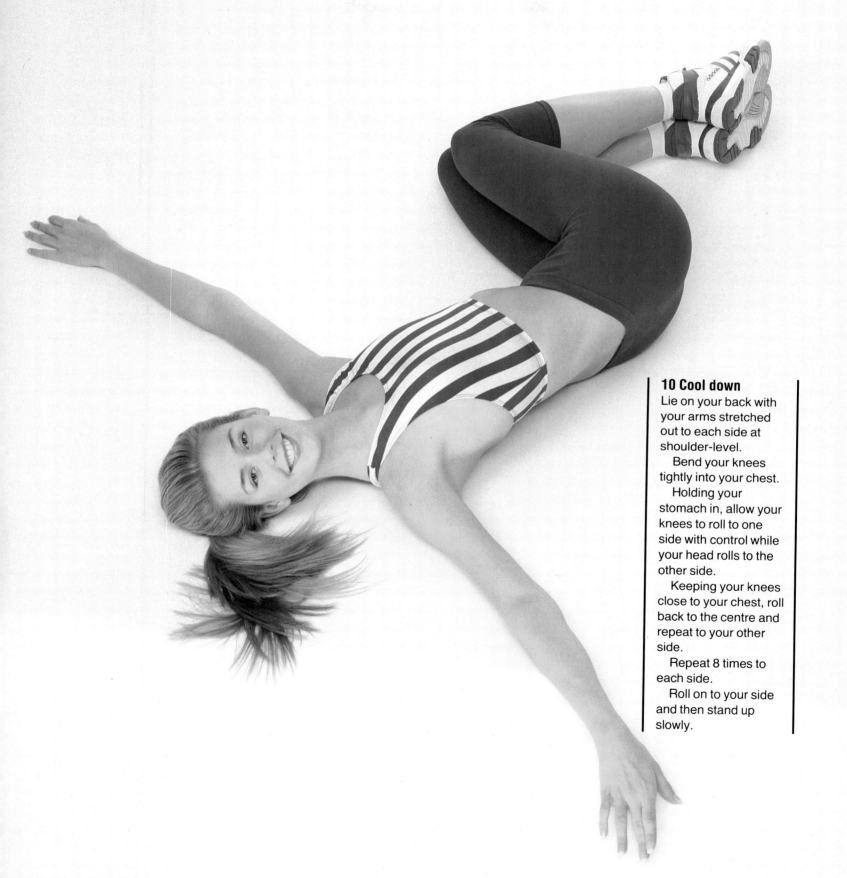

10 Cool down
Lie on your back with your arms stretched out to each side at shoulder-level.

Bend your knees tightly into your chest.

Holding your stomach in, allow your knees to roll to one side with control while your head rolls to the other side.

Keeping your knees close to your chest, roll back to the centre and repeat to your other side.

Repeat 8 times to each side.

Roll on to your side and then stand up slowly.

STRESSED OUT

Identify the sources of stress in your daily life and then stress-proof your environment with these easy tricks.

Stress – that feeling of pressure – sets off a chain reaction of disturbances in the body. Extra adrenalin rushes round (this is part of the body's defence system to give you energy in a crisis). The nervous system is stimulated, hormone production altered, muscles tense up, white blood cells produce fewer antibodies and acid production is increased in the digestive organs. These internal changes give us outward signs of stress.

Stress signals
- irritability, headaches, anxiety
- fatigue, coupled with difficulty in actually getting to sleep
- mood swings, sudden outbursts, indecision
- loss of libido, lack of interest or enjoyment in life
- increased incidence of spots – adult acne has been linked to stress
- vulnerability to illness and flare-ups of existing conditions such as ezcema and herpes
- digestive problems
- undereating, overeating, binge-eating
- hair loss – stress is a major cause of female hair loss
- trembling and other nervous reflexes.

Everyone is vulnerable to stress. Its causes are manifold and include relationship problems, bereavement, moving house and a high-pressure job, but we all have different tolerance levels.

One theory psychologists have put forward to explain why people react differently to stress is that stress is related to personality type.
- The 'type A' personality is typically impatient, speaks fast and loudly, is ambitious and always in a hurry, with a tendency to try and do a number of things at the same time, such as working and eating.
- The 'type B' personality is altogether much calmer, taking life at a slower pace with a more relaxed and easy-going approach.

While we are mostly a *mixture* of the two types, we tend to exhibit more characteristics of one or the other. Type A is more stress-prone and thus more at risk of stress-related disease, such as a heart attack, than type B.

Protecting yourself from stress
There are certain steps you can take to guard against stress.
- Make time for relaxation and leave work at work.
- Keep rhythm in your life, as the body responds well to routine. Try, particularly to establish sleep patterns, that is, go to bed and wake up at the same time each day.
- Be aware of what may be causing your stress and try to sort out the problem, or at least anticipate it. Get support from others – suffering in silence doesn't help.
- Prioritize and do only what is important. What wouldn't bother you in a few months or years really isn't worth worrying about.
- Eat a healthy, balanced diet.
- Take some form of exercise three times a week and make it a habit. Exercise is a great antidote to stress, because it lowers your blood pressure and releases endorphins, the body's own natural mood-enhancing chemicals.

DAILY DE-STRESSORS
There are many recurring sources of stress that are part of the regular pattern of your life. It helps to be aware of them when you are aiming to reduce your stress levels.

Stress at the desk
Often, it is at work that you feel at your most 'stressed out'. Colleagues' demands, the constant ringing of telephones and a heavy workload can add up to pressure that at times may seem too much.

Don't panic! Close your eyes and count slowly back from 50. You should be feeling calmer already.

Read on and discover other ways to stress-proof your workspace.

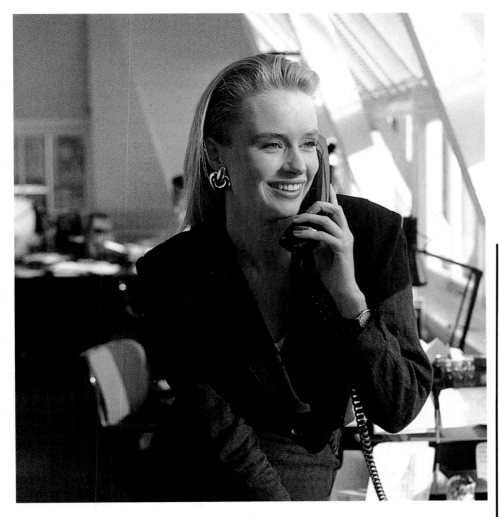

Stress-proofing tips
● Check your posture while you are sitting at your desk. You should be sitting up straight, with your bottom into the back of the chair, with your shoulders down and back, and your chest forward.

It is a natural reaction to let your posture go when you are under stress, so that your shoulders are slumped forward and your head sinks into your neck. In this position, you're setting yourself up for aches and pains and will also be breathing incorrectly.

Try sitting up straight with your head facing forwards – place two fingers on your chin and 'push' back in towards your neck until your head feels balanced and your neck long instead of curved.
● When working at a VDU or reading lots of small print, look into the distance or close your eyes for a few minutes from time to time to avoid or ease eye strain.
● Don't cradle the phone between your shoulder and chin. It will lead to headaches, neck and upper back pain and possibly 'telephone acne' on the chin.

Use your hands to hold the receiver and switch it from ear to ear and, as a preventive measure against spots, clean the mouthpiece daily.
● Do quick exercises during the day to avoid neck strain and relax your shoulders (see page 24).

STRESS AND YOUR DIET
A regular, balanced diet keeps your body in optimum health. During times of stress – whether short-term or prolonged – it is even more important to watch what you eat, as stress is a nutrient robber. See page 12 for general advice, but bear in mind the following points.
● Vitamin C is used at a faster rate when you are under stress, so increase your fruit and vegetable intake, especially raw fruit and vegetables as some vitamin C is lost during cooking.
● When you are under stress you may find yourself craving sugar as a comforter. Carbohydrates have actually been found to trigger a calming chemical in the brain, soothing negative feelings, anxiety and anger. Although you may want refined carbohydrates such as chocolate, choose complex carbohydrates such as pasta, crackers and grains instead. These will give you a more prolonged feeling of calm, rather than the quick 'up', followed by a deep low that refined carbohydrates induce.
● Avoid drinking lots of stimulating tea and coffee, which, like refined carbohydrates will make you go faster temporarily, but bring you down with a thud a little later. Opt for mineral water, juice and herb teas instead.

STRESS-BEATING RELAXATION

Calm your mind and revitalize your body with our instant stress-reducing strategies.

If, in spite of all your efforts to eliminate sources of stress from your life, you still become tense and anxious, there are many ways to deal with it.

SLEEPING IT OFF

Restful sleep is one of the best reliefs for stress. However, you may find that your stress is causing disturbed sleep patterns or creating problems with actually getting to sleep. Try these tips.

Before bed-time . . .
● Avoid stimulants such as tea, coffee and nicotine.
● Beware alcohol – it may make you *feel* sleepy at first, but it tends to create a fitful sleep, making you wake up at frequent intervals.
● Try a relaxing bath, listening to soothing music.
● Gentle stretching exercises are good before bedtime, but don't undertake aerobic activity as it stimulates the cardio-vascular and nervous systems for up to six hours afterwards.
● If you've got a problem, try to solve it *before* going to bed or leave it and vow you'll sort it out in the morning.

In bed . . . and still not asleep?
● Try some Autogenic Training – a relaxation technique that uses

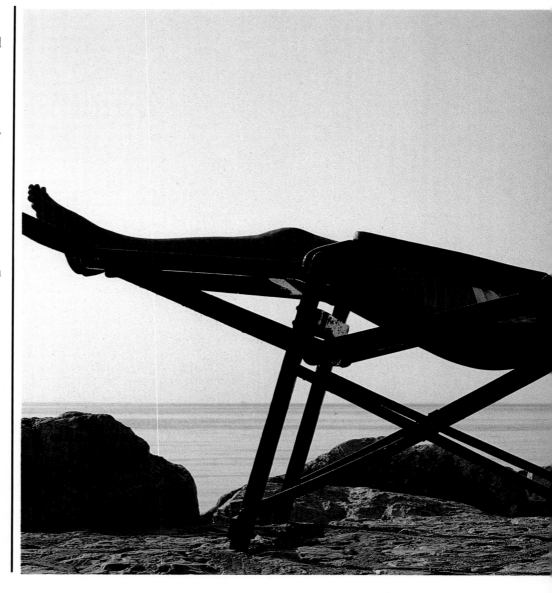

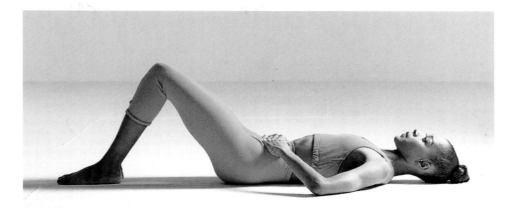

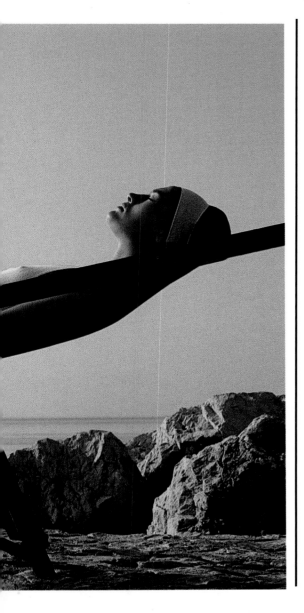

conditioned responses to imagery to control bodily tension. Concentrate on how heavy, sleepy and warm your body feels, imagining all the muscles and limbs from head to toe.

● Counting sheep or visualizing a black space helps because it is meaningless and diverts your mind from your troubles.

● As a last resort, try a diversionary tactic like getting up and reading or watching TV.

MEDITATING

Soothe yourself with meditation – it's a valuable de-stressing technique that works well for many people.

A simple method of meditating is to sit quietly for a few minutes and repeat a word you have positive associations with, either out loud or in your head.

Alternatively, there's the progressive muscle relaxation method. Take ten minutes out, first tensing and then relaxing your muscle groups, starting with the muscles at the feet and working your way up through all the parts of the body to the neck area.

Relaxation tapes also have de-stressing benefits. They feature a calming voice talking to you, giving you muscle relaxation techniques to follow and helping you visualize a calmer you.

BREATHING

We rarely think about how we breathe, we simply do it. However, nine times out of ten, we are doing it incorrectly – breathing too shallowly and irregularly. Incorrect breathing can cause tension, panic attacks and lack of concentration. Conscious deep breathing is calming and increases circulation. It reduces toxic build-ups in the body, eliminating excess carbon dioxide to keep the blood pH levels and the nervous system stable.

Shallow breathing from the chest only is common when we are tense and stressed. To breathe correctly, check your posture and relax your stomach. Inhale deeply from the abdomen, drawing the diaphragm down and exhale with the same control.

Practice this simple breathing exercise every day. During the exercise your fingers should separate as a result of abdominal expansion.

● Lie on your back on the floor with your knees bent, feet flat on the floor. Put your hands on your stomach, palms on hips, fingers just touching in the middle.

● Exhale through your mouth, and pull your navel in, for a count of 4.

● Hold for 4 and then inhale through your nose, to a count of 4.

● Repeat five times.

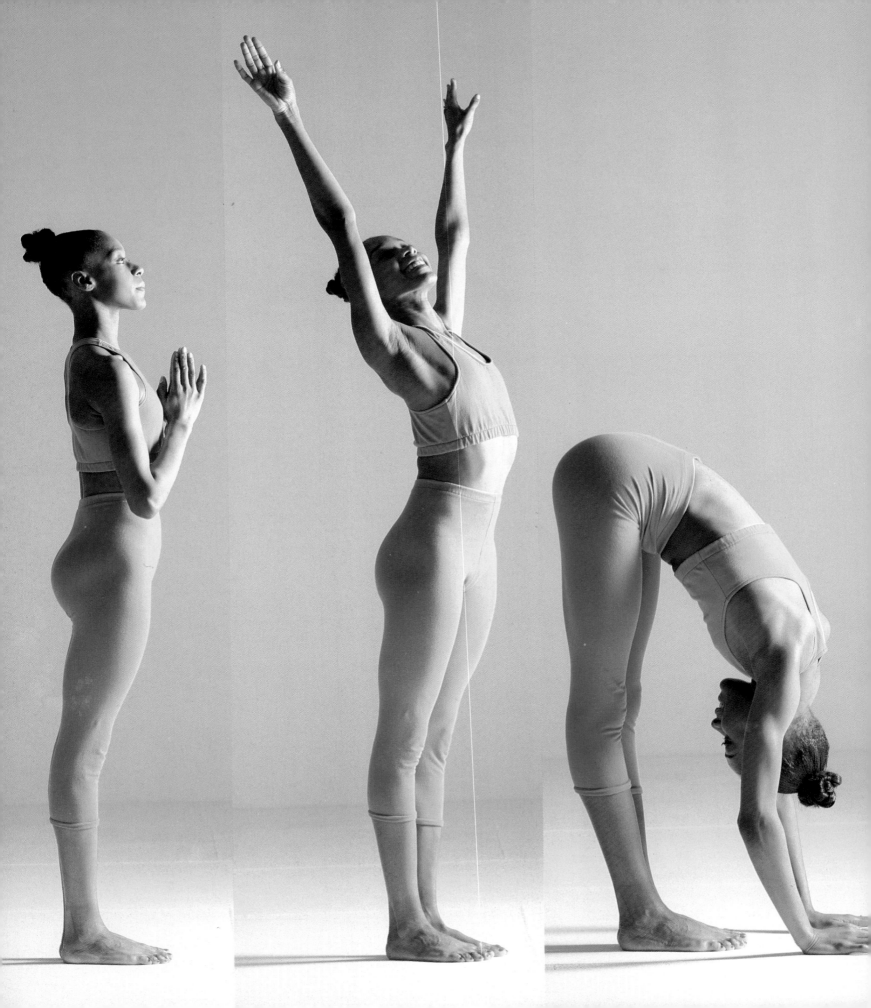

SALUTE TO THE SUN

Face the day feeling refreshed and ready for anything with this energizing yoga sequence.

Yoga uses stretching techniques to tone and revitalize the body. It's a mind-led discipline, very controlled and particularly beneficial for correcting posture.

While attending classes to learn correct techniques is advisable, the sequence shown here, the 'Salute to the Sun', is easy to master. It is a routine ideally suited to the morning. It will energize you and make you feel calm and ready for the day.

Do the moves as a flowing sequence, breathing in as you bend back and exhaling when you are bending forwards. If it is comfortable, hold each position for up to 10 seconds.

1 Stand up straight with your feet together. Tuck your pelvis under, taking care not to hollow your back. With your hands together, breathe slowly in and out.

2 While breathing deeply, stretch your arms out in front and arch them over your head so you are leaning back slightly. Bring your arms forwards again and breathe out.

3 *Bending your knees* if you are not very flexible, lean over from the waist. Tuck your head in. Stretch as far as you can keeping your knees bent.

4 In a sweeping movement, bend one knee underneath you, foot flat on the floor, with your other leg stretched out behind you. Keep your hands on the ground and look up, while breathing in. Sweep back into the position described in the third step, breathe again, and flow into the position described at the beginning of this step, reversing the leg movement.

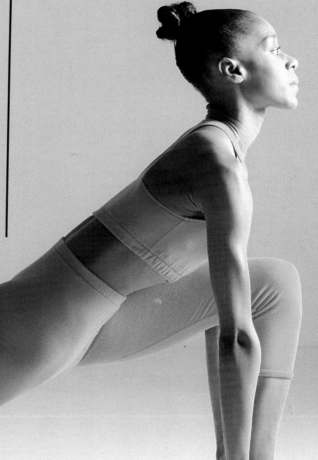

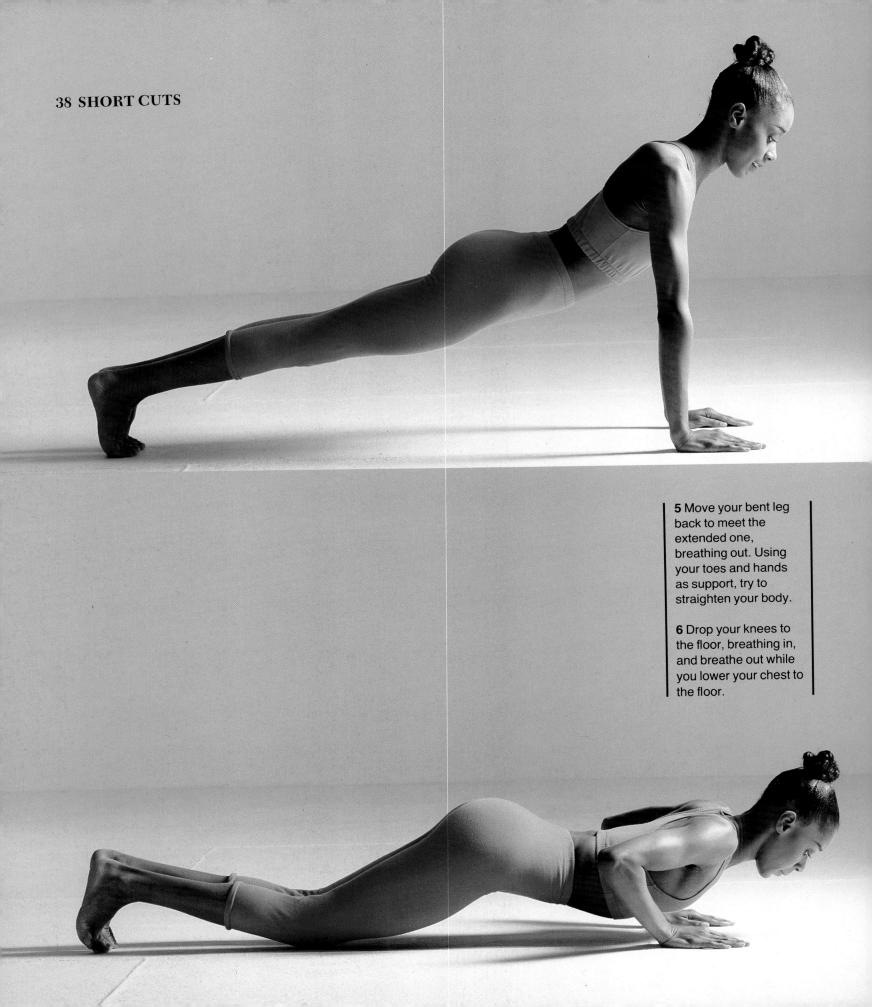

5 Move your bent leg back to meet the extended one, breathing out. Using your toes and hands as support, try to straighten your body.

6 Drop your knees to the floor, breathing in, and breathe out while you lower your chest to the floor.

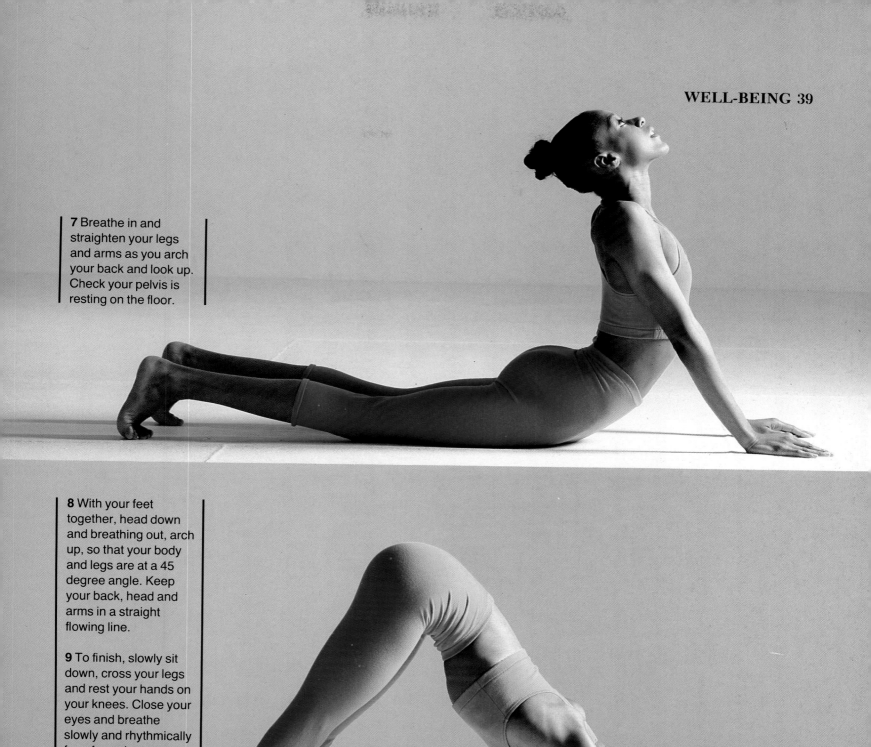

7 Breathe in and straighten your legs and arms as you arch your back and look up. Check your pelvis is resting on the floor.

8 With your feet together, head down and breathing out, arch up, so that your body and legs are at a 45 degree angle. Keep your back, head and arms in a straight flowing line.

9 To finish, slowly sit down, cross your legs and rest your hands on your knees. Close your eyes and breathe slowly and rhythmically for a few minutes. Open your eyes and stand up slowly.

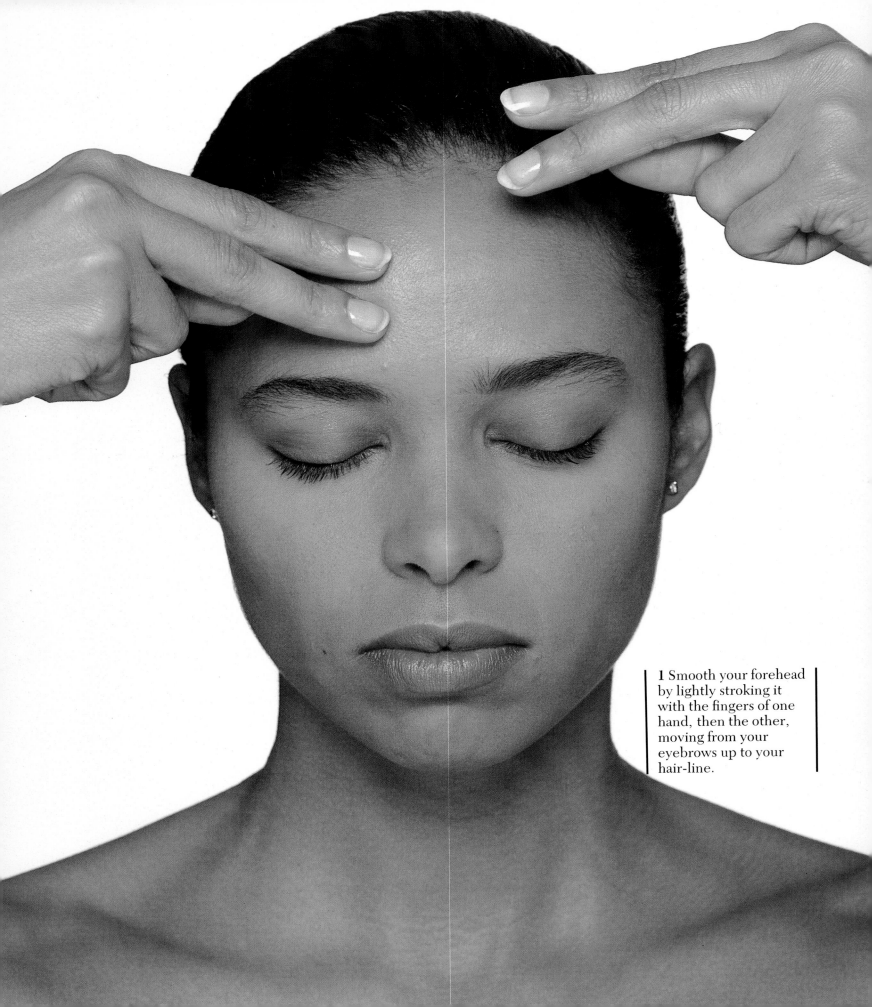

1 Smooth your forehead by lightly stroking it with the fingers of one hand, then the other, moving from your eyebrows up to your hair-line.

MARVELLOUS MASSAGE

You can ease away tension, revive your skin and increase circulation by using the simplest massage techniques.

Massage has been used for centuries to relax the body and soothe the mind. Many people are taking weekend or evening courses in massage techniques to discover more about the power of massage and to learn the basic methods. In fact, massage is as enjoyable and relaxing for the masseur as it is for the person receiving the treatment.

Simply massaging your upper arms and shoulders when you feel fatigued and tense will help to keep circulation moving and prevent problems. Squeeze and release the skin firmly, moving up the arm and across the shoulders using the hand of the opposite arm. Concentrate on areas where you can feel tight, knotted muscles.

FACIAL MASSAGE
This is another fast way to ease out lines created by tiredness and stress. The gentle massaging movements of your fingers will immediately make you feel calmer and more relaxed. It increases the microcirculation and thereby improves the colour and condition of your complexion.

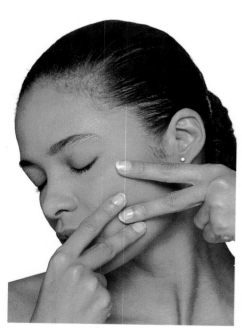

2 Make small scissor movements all over your face, using the first two fingers of both hands, lightly pulling and pushing your fingers together in an interlocking V-shape.

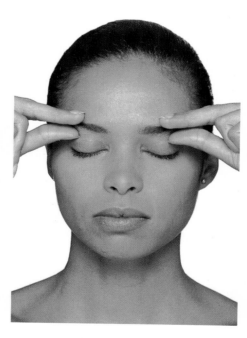

3 Pinch your eyebrows, from your nose out to your temples, using your thumbs and index fingers.

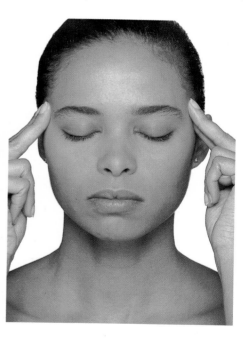

4 With the pads of your fingers at your temples, sit quietly with your eyes closed and circle your fingers slowly 6 times. Press your temples, hold for 5 seconds and repeat.

AROMATIC ENERGY

Aromatherapy oils bring immediate improvement to everyday health and beauty problems. Discover the power of these potent plant remedies.

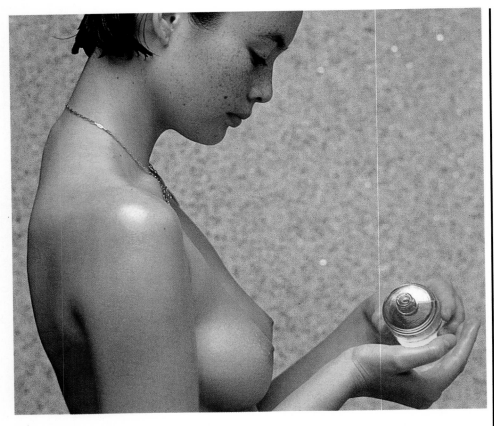

Aromatherapy is rapidly growing in popularity, as a result of its ability to improve our sense of well-being and to treat a wide variety of everyday health complaints. It was used by the Egyptians and came to the fore again this century when physicians researched the subject in depth. It is now widely practised in Great Britain, France and other countries.

Aromatherapy uses essential oils, the distilled essences of herbs and plants which have therapeutic properties and a wonderful scent. Essential oils work on two levels: they can revive us emotionally and psychologically because the aromatic molecules have a direct pathway to the brain via the olfactory system. They work physically by entering the skin and aromatherapists claim, travelling through the bloodstream.

You can buy the oils from health shops and specialist outlets. It is worth buying highest quality oils. Aromatherapy products prepared in advance are also available. There are a number of ways to use essential oils at home.

● Try them in the bath, adding approximately six drops and swirling the water around with your hand before getting in. Close the bathroom door and inhale the stress-relieving aroma.

● You can also inhale essential oils by placing six to ten drops in a basin of hot water and then placing a towel over your head and the basin. This method is useful if you have a cold, headache or are under stress. Many essential oils are anti-viral and antiseptic.

● A massage with plant essences is a wonderful treat. Use two drops of your chosen oil to 10 ml (2 teaspoons) of a carrier oil, such as sunflower or almond.

Note that essential oils should not be applied neat to the skin in most instances as they are very concentrated.

● Spritz your home and office with the oils. Place a drop in a plant spray filled with water and spray into the atmosphere.

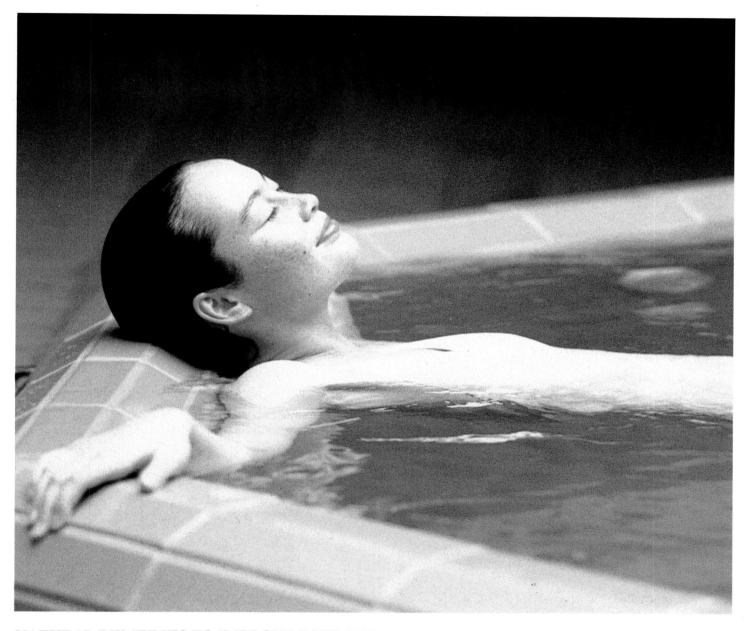

NATURAL REMEDIES TO IMPROVE YOUR WELL-BEING
These common health problems can be eased by the use of the following oils.

Anxiety	Cellulite	Colds	Headaches	PMT
Use the oils in any of the ways described opposite.	Use the oils for massage or in a bath.	Inhale the oils, add them to your bath or spray them into the atmosphere.	Use the oils as for colds.	Use the oils in any of the ways described opposite; massage is particularly good.
Camomile	Cypress	Basil	Lavender	Geranium
Clary Sage	Fennel	Eucalyptus	Peppermint	Lavender
Geranium	Geranium	Majoram	Rosemary	Neroli
Lavender	Juniper	Tea Tree	Thyme	Rose
Rose	Sage			

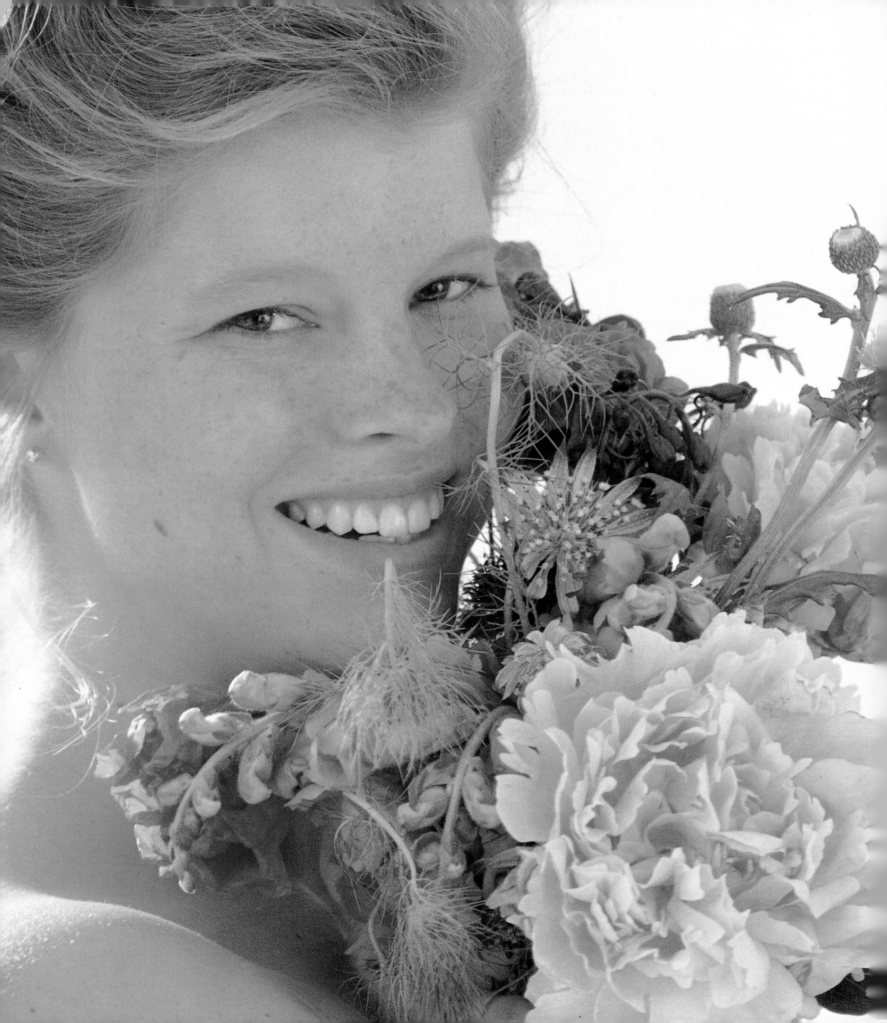

SKINCARE

What you do – or don't do – to your skin will be reflected in its condition today and in the years to come. It is not necessary to follow a complicated routine and, in fact, simple skincare is best. With our special quick-to-do programmes and vital tips, maintaining your skin in prime condition is easy – however short on time you may be.

SKIN TYPING

*Finding your skin type is the key to developing
an effective skincare programme.*

Knowing a little about the structure of your skin will help you appreciate why certain things are good for it and others are not. Understand your skin and you are halfway to a glowing, healthy complexion.

The skin is formed from three main layers: the epidermis, dermis and hypodermis.

The epidermis is the outermost layer and is just a microscopic 0.2 mm (8/1000 in) thick on the face. The surface consists of dead cells which are in the process of flaking away and new ones which are growing to take their place. Between the epidermis and dermis lies the basal layer, where new epidermal cells are formed and progress to the surface. It takes approximately twenty-eight days for a new cell to reach the top.

The dermis is usually about 1.8 mm (7/100 in) thick. It is composed of a fibrous protein called collagen, elastin, which makes the skin supple, and a network of blood vessels, nerves, oil and sweat glands, pores and hair follicles.

The hypodermis is the tissue beneath both the epidermis and the dermis. It contains muscles, veins and fat cells and its thickness varies according to the part of the body.

The sebum and sweat produced by the oil and sweat glands in the dermis form a hydro-lipidic film on

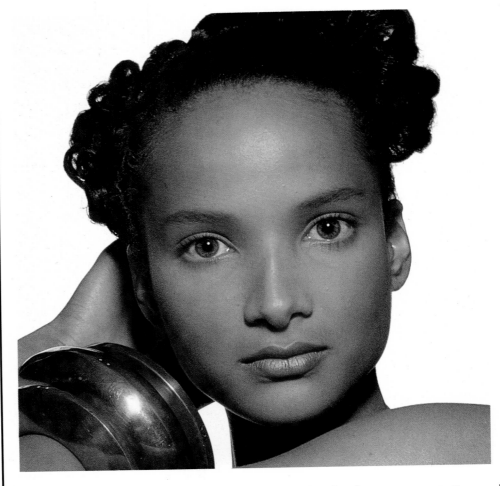

the skin. This film, known as the 'acid mantle', lubricates the skin's surface, helps to repel bacteria and protects against irritation. The acid mantle maintains the skin's slightly acid pH level. It takes one to two

hours for the skin to return to its normal pH level after washing. Using harsh cleansers, such as soaps, reduces the ability of the skin to renew the acid mantle.

It is the activity of the sebaceous

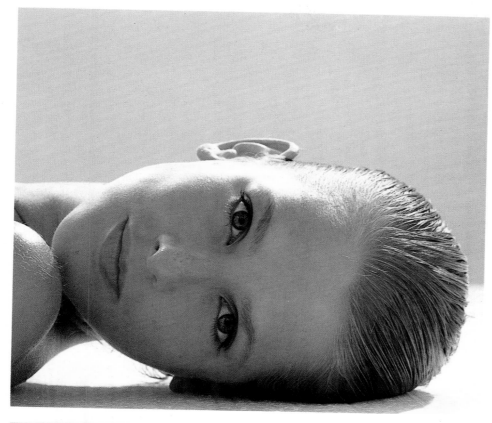

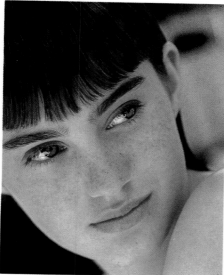

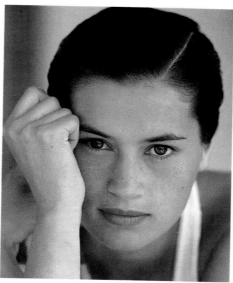

IDENTIFY YOUR SKIN TYPE

By answering the questions below you can find out what type of skin you have. Just tick the answer – a, b, c or d – that most closely applies to your skin.

1 **After cleansing, how does your skin feel?**
   a Tight and rough.
   b Smooth and supple.
   c Slightly oily.
   d Oily in some areas, tight in others.

2 **How often does your skin break out in spots?**
   a Almost never.
   b Rarely.
   c Often.
   d Only in the T-zone.

3 **Which of the following best describes your skin texture?**
   a Smooth and transparent.
   b Firm and even.
   c Slightly rough and uneven.
   d A mixture of the above.

4 **How does your skin look during the day?**
   a Flaky and chapped.
   b Clean and fresh-looking.
   c Shiny.
   d Shiny in the T-zone.

Now, add up how many a's, b's, c's and d's you scored.

If the majority of your answers are a's, your skin is dry.
If the majority of your answers are b's, your skin is normal.
If the majority of your answers are c's, your skin is oily.
If the majority of your answers are d's, your skin is combination.

(oil-producing) glands that determine your skin type. Activity in the T-zone (across the forehead and down the nose and chin) may be greater than elsewhere.

There are four main skin types: dry, normal, oily and combination, although 'normal' skin often tends towards oily or dry. Within these groups there are skins that require special attention, such as sensitive skins and black skins.

PERFECT YOUR SKIN

Choosing the right type of cleanser, toner and moisturizer is the key to the healthiest, clearest skin.

The skin responds best to a regular routine, which can be quick but must be a discipline. Now that you have found out your skin type, learn the best cleansing and moisturizing system for you.

CLEANSING

This is a top priority if you want to have good skin. A quick cleanse in the morning (to remove toxins that have reached the surface via the sweat glands) and a thorough cleanse at night are important for every skin type. Soap doesn't remove make-up and can be drying, so use soap-free cleansing bars, or wash-off or wipe-off cleansing creams instead.

Toner, or freshener, removes the last traces of dirt and excess cleanser. Some toners contain alcohol to remove excess oil, but alcohol-free toners are a better choice. Toner containing alcohol can be drying and should be diluted even for oily skins.

Removing eye make-up
● Dab a little eye make-up remover on to two cotton wool pads.
● Using one pad for each eye (to avoid the spread of infection), hold it against your lashes for a few seconds to dissolve the make-up.
● Supporting the skin by placing the fingers of your opposite hand on your brow, stroke in towards your nose and down from your eyebrow. Don't move the pad up and out as you will pull the skin in the wrong direction.

Using wipe-off cleanser
● Warm the cleanser in your hands so that it doesn't go on cold.
● Smooth it over your face with your whole hand, starting at the neck and working up and out.
● Place your thumbs under your chin and work the cleanser in little circles with your index fingers around your nose and chin.
● Remove the cleanser by wiping it off gently with a soft tissue or a piece of cotton wool.

Using wash-off cleanser
● Dampen the skin with warm water and use the same movements given above to apply the cleanser.
● Rinse the cleanser off very thoroughly with comfortably warm running water. Water that is too hot will dehydrate the skin and cause broken capillaries.
● Pat your face dry with a tissue or a clean towel.

Using toner
● Sweep the toner on to your face with a cotton wool pad, moving up and out, avoiding the eye area.
● Blot your skin dry with a tissue.

MOISTURIZING

Moisturizers are formulated to tackle different skin problems.

Creams help balance drier skin, while lotions and emulsions are designed for normal to oily complexions. Innovative, featherweight formulations are the lastest trend – containing high-powered hydrating ingredients, they are suitable for every skin type. Oil-free and gel moisturizers are perfect for oily complexions. Anti-ageing ingredients and nutrients, such as vitamins, are often added to help improve cell turnover and oxygenation of the tissues. Night creams are useful from the age of twenty-five, especially for dry skins, but avoid very heavy creams as these can result in puffiness.

Moisturizing the very delicate skin surrounding the eyes calls for special products. Your usual moisturizer may cause puffiness and stretch the skin. Eye gel is wonderfully refreshing in the morning, and a little eye cream will strengthen the tissues at night. Pat on either, using the third and fourth fingers, tapping quickly but gently.

Your usual moisturizer is fine for your neck, although a product specially formulated for this area, which is so susceptible to ageing, makes good beauty sense.

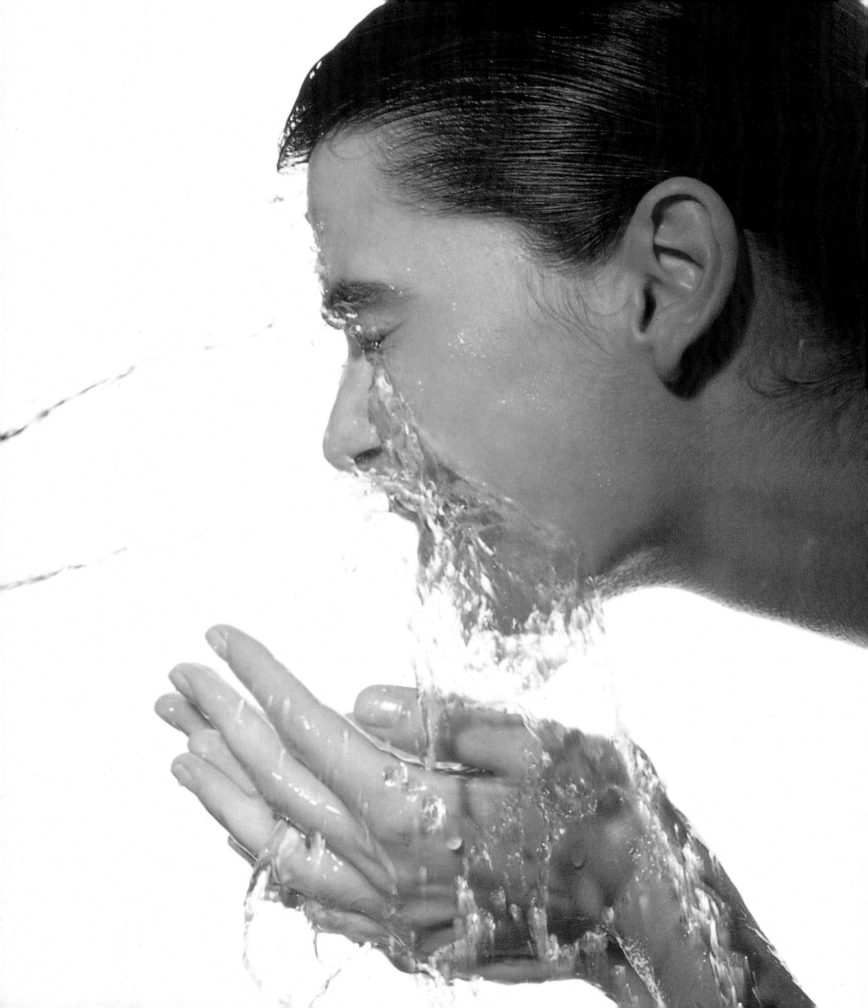

QUICK SKINCARE SYSTEMS

Customizing your skincare products to your skin type is easy with these 5-minute skincare programmes.

DRY SKIN

- *It has a fine, matte texture.*
- *It may be on the sensitive side.*
- *There are usually no visible or open pores.*
- *It is more prone to fine lines and wrinkles than other skin types.*
- *It is more vulnerable to the effects of central heating and sunlight.*
- *Very fair skin is often dry.*

5-minute skincare

Morning
- Cleanse quickly, using a wipe-off cleanser for dry skin.
- Tone, using alcohol-free toner on water-moistened cotton wool.
- Hydrate with a moisturizer for dry skin, preferably one containing a broad-spectrum sunscreen. Avoid your eyes.

Evening
- Remove your eye make-up.
- Cleanse as above, but more thoroughly.
- Apply a night cream.

NORMAL SKIN

One hundred per cent normal skin is a rare blessing.
- *It is smooth textured with no visible pores.*
- *It shows no signs of dryness in youth.*
- *It has an even tone that is not too pale, sallow or red.*
- *It will tend towards dryness with age and as a result of external influences.*

5-minute skincare

Morning
- Cleanse using a wipe-off or wash-off cleanser for normal-to-dry skin.
- Tone using alcohol-free toner on a water-moistened cotton ball.
- Hydrate with a moisturizer for normal skin.

Evening
- Remove your eye make-up first, then cleanse as above, but more thoroughly.
- Apply moisturizer or a lightweight night lotion.

OILY SKIN

- *It has open pores.*
- *It will shine an hour or so after washing.*
- *It may look oily on waking.*
- *It has a tendency to spots and blackheads.*
- *It is less susceptible to wrinkles than other skin types.*

5-minute skincare

Morning
- Cleanse quickly using a wipe-off cleanser for normal-to-oily skin or a soap-free cleansing bar. Rinse very thoroughly.
- Tone using a toner that should be diluted if it contains alcohol so that it is not too drying. Moisten your cotton wool with water.
- Moisturize where needed using an oil-free or gel moisturizer.

Evening
- Remove eye make-up, then cleanse as above, but more thoroughly.
- Apply moisturizer just where needed.

COMBINATION SKIN

- *The centre T-zone (across the forehead and down the nose and chin) is oily and coarser in texture than the rest of the skin, and may have a tendency to spots or blackheads.*
- *The cheeks are normal or even dry.*

5-minute skincare

Morning
- Cleanse quickly using a wipe-off cleanser for normal-to-oily skins.
- Tone, using a toner without alcohol.
- Moisturize just where needed using an oil-free or gel moisturizer.

Evening
- Remove your eye make-up, then cleanse as above, but more thoroughly and concentrate on the T-zone.
- Use a moisturizer or night cream on dry areas only, particularly the cheeks.

SENSITIVE SKIN

- *Looks fragile and translucent.*
- *It is generally dry.*
- *It may have freckles.*
- *It tends to become flushed, blotchy and irritated in extremes of temperature or through using harsh cleansing products.*
- *It may suffer from broken red veins, dermatitis, allergies.*

5-minute skincare

Follow the programme for dry skin.

Special tips

- Look for hypo-allergenic products that are fragrance and lanolin-free.
- Before trying a new product do a patch test. Rub a good amount on to your shoulder and leave it on overnight. If there is no sign of irritation, apply some to your neck and wait again. If there is no reaction then the product will probably be safe to use on your face.

BLACK SKIN

● *Tends towards extremes of oiliness or dryness which can be a real problem since these conditions are more visible against a darker complexion. Dry black skin may appear greyish in colour.*

● *It needs very gentle care as face scrubs, spots, ear piercing and hair removal can make the supply of melanin uneven, leading to skin that is darker or lighter in some places than others.*

5-minute skincare
Follow the programme for dry or oily skins.

Special tips
● If your skin is sensitive use toners that do not contain alcohol, and fragrance-free products.
● If flaky, grey-looking skin is a problem, gently use a flannel to slough the skin, or use a peel-off mask.

OLIVE SKIN

● *It tends towards oiliness and often has larger pores.*
● *Any sallowness is due to the lack of pink pigment.*

5-minute skincare
Follow the programme for oily skins.

A MIXTURE OF SKIN TYPES
Skin may develop the characteristics of several skin types as a result of incorrect treatment and environmental skin hazards. For example:

● *An oily, spotty skin can also suffer from the dry skin problems of fine surface lines and flaking if you work in an over-heated office, perhaps smoke or eat a poor diet, or use harsh and abrasive cleaners (over-enthusiastic scrubbing with anti-bacterial products can aggravate oily skin and dry the surface).*

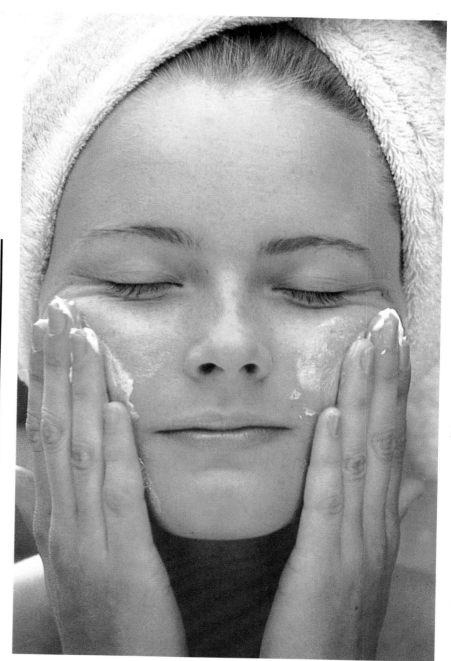

● *A skin that is usually dry can develop small bumps under the skin and spots as a result of a poor diet, insufficient cleansing or using a skin cream that is too rich.*

FAST SKIN BOOSTERS

Get your skin glowing with fast and easy treatments you can do at home.

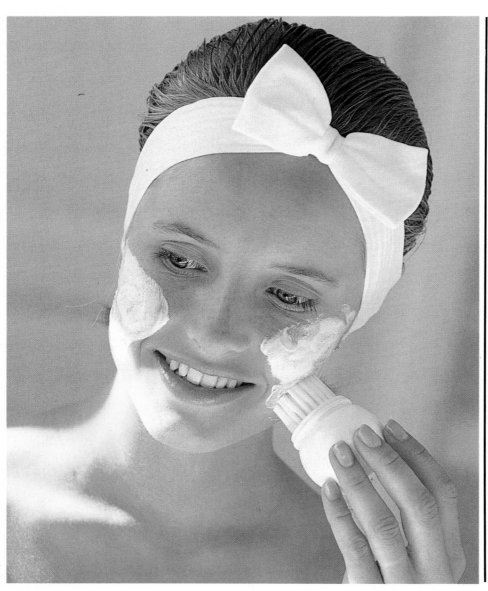

EXFOLIATION

Exfoliators, or skin sloughers, are speedy skin improvers. By removing the dead cells from the surface of the skin, face 'scrubs' make your skin smoother and brighter in seconds. They also help skin that is prone to spots stay clearer and increase the cell turnover so the skin looks younger for longer.

It is important to choose a product that is very gentle so that the grains do not scratch the skin.

Tips for using an exfoliator

- Use a facial scrub on cleansed, damp skin.
- Rest your thumb against your skin (this ensures that you don't use the full power of your arm) and use very light, circular movements.
- Never rub your skin until it changes colour and do not use exfoliators near your eyes.
- If your skin is fair, sensitive or very fine, use a peel-off mask instead of a facial scrub to lift away dead cells and revitalize your complexion.
- Exfoliation is very useful for black skin, which can look ashen in colour, but a peel-off mask is better than a face scrub, as black skin is vulnerable to changes in pigmentation and face scrubs can trigger this.

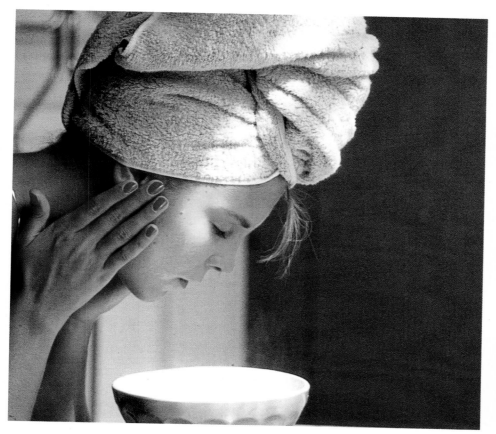

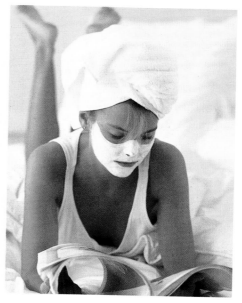

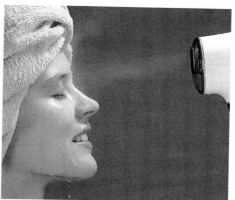

• Although facial scrubs help prevent your skin breaking out in spots, do not use them if your skin is already inflamed or infected as you may spread the infection. This is true for the body, too.

MARVELLOUS MASKS

Masks are a really good way to pep up skin in no time at all.

Cleansing masks, which often contain clay or fruit, absorb excess oils. The enzymes in fruits such as papaya have a deep-cleansing action and leave the skin glowing.

Moisturizing masks give drier skin a real boost, smoothing out fine lines and refreshing the face. Some moisturizing masks also contain toning and firming ingredients, such as seaweed, herbs and aromatherapy oils and are excellent as complexion-improvers before a party or after a late night.

STEAMING

Steaming is an effective way of cleansing the skin. You can add herbs, such as soothing camomile.

If you have sensitive skin or skin that is prone to broken capillaries, however, specialists recommend that you do not cleanse with steam.

Tips for steaming

• Cleanse your skin first.
• Pour water that is almost boiling into a bowl and lean over the steam. Draping a towel over your head and the bowl will prevent steam escaping.
• Be very careful not to get too close to the water (stay 30 cm, 12 in or so away). Do not steam for more than a few minutes.
• Apply a cleansing mask afterwards, while your skin is still warm, or cleanse your skin again and massage moisturizer into it.

EARLY MORNING SKIN WAKE-UPS

To revive a pallid complexion try the following quick tricks:

• *Spritz your skin with cool water from a mini plant spray kept in the refrigerator. Replenish it frequently with fresh water. Pat your skin gently and moisturize while it is still slightly damp.*
• *Alternatively, cleanse your skin quickly and apply a moisturizing mask before you have breakfast or get dressed. Then remove the mask and apply a tinted moisturizer.*
• *Go out for a brisk walk in the fresh air.*

FABULOUS FACIALS

For a luxurious beauty boost, expert care and advice, try a salon facial precisely tailored to your skin's needs.

Having a facial at a beauty salon can bring immediate improvement to many skin conditions and give the complexion a fresh new look. Dryness that is due to sunbathing or the ageing process for instance, acne and blackheads, or a skin that lacks vitality, are some of the problems that can be helped.

The bonus of a salon facial is that the therapist has in-depth training and can advise you as to whether your skin is in good condition for your age, bearing in mind your life-style. She will choose products to treat individual areas of the face and can combine several types of treatments to tend precisely to your skin's needs. These treatments include the following:

Steaming This warms and softens the skin, making it easier to remove blackheads.

Massage Many therapists believe that this is the most important element of a facial. A beauty therapist may massage for up to 20 minutes, focusing on key acupressure points. Massaging the skin increases the skin's micro-circulation and improves lymphatic drainage. Lymph is a natural fluid produced by the lymph glands and acts as the body's waste disposal system: unlike blood, lymph does not have a 'pump' to circulate it but

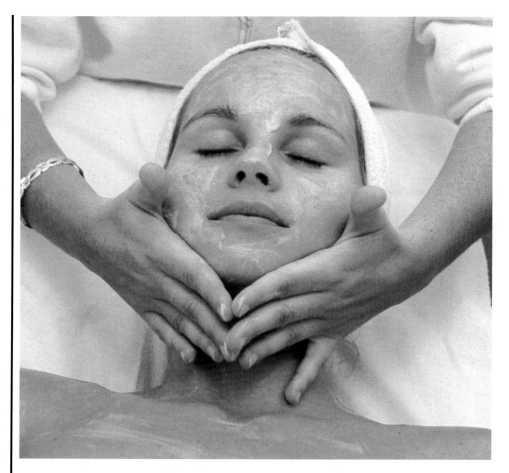

relies on muscle activity to move it around the body.

Because of the complicated bone structure in the face the lymph can become congested here, causing a tired-looking complexion that may be prone to spots.

Galvanic current Using gels chosen according to skin type, the therapist applies galvanic current via a roller. The gel is drawn into the pores and causes perspiration, thereby removing grime. The treatment is completely painless!

High frequency A tube which carries electric current sparks inside as it is moved over the face by the therapist. This sterilizes the skin with ozone, bathes the skin in oxygen and stimulates cell turnover. This too is painless.

Ampoule treatment Very concentrated, active ingredients contained in sealed glass phials, or ampoules, are massaged into the skin. The seal ensures the ingredients remain fresh. Extracts of herbs, royal jelly, wheatgerm, vitamins and collagen are some of the elements used for their intensive and fast-acting results. Although collagen has been found to have too large a molecule to penetrate the skin, it is used for its softening and moisturizing effect.

Alternative therapies Many beauty therapists are now trained in alternative medicine and may use a technique such as auricular therapy (massage of key points on the ears) or reflexology (oriental foot and hand massage, where the therapist massages areas of the feet and hands which relate to specific areas of the face and body) to improve general health and the condition of the skin.

Aromatherapy facials using essential oils from plants are very popular. As well as using them for massage or a mask, the therapist may add them to the steamer.

How often should you have a facial?
Once a month is ideal for most skins, although neglected or problem skins may require attention once a week until the skin shows improvement. If you cannot afford the time and money every month, it is a good idea to go to a salon at the change of a season so that you can check your skincare routine is on the right track.

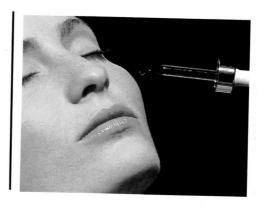

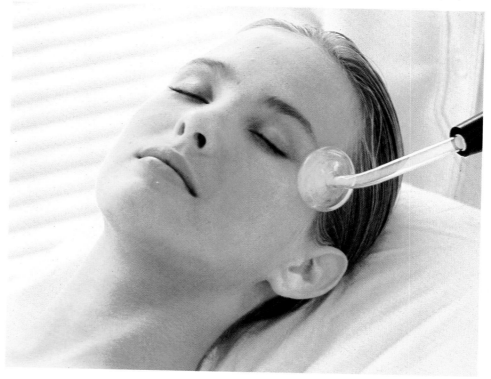

ANTI-AGEING STRATEGIES

Keep your skin looking young with simple precautions you can easily incorporate into your daily life.

Protecting and caring for your skin today will, without doubt, benefit you in the years to come. While hereditary factors play a crucial role in determining how well your skin will age, there are many preventive measures you can take that will help to keep your skin glowing and keep wrinkles at bay.

Protection from the sun
Dermatologists all agree that sun is the prime ager of skin. Sunbathing without protection causes breakdown of collagen, dehydration of the skin tissues, thickening of the skin texture and, ultimately, wrinkles.

Skin protection tip
Wearing moisturizers with built-in sunscreens *year-round*, even in temperate climates, is being increasingly recommended as an anti-ageing strategy.

These dual-purpose moisturizers are one of the best short cuts to keeping your skin in perfect condition.

Regular skincare
A cleansing and moisturizing programme that you follow daily is an essential anti-ageing strategy. It has been scientifically proven that dehydrated skin is more likely to develop wrinkles.

Constant eyecare
Wrinkles around the eyes cannot be avoided altogether, but you can strengthen the skin in this delicate area by cleansing very carefully. Do not pull the skin the wrong way when removing eye make-up. Stroke the pad of remover in towards your nose and down from your brow, not away. Use special eye products.

Exercise
Exercising regularly has many positive effects on your skin:
● It makes it glow by stimulating blood circulation and increasing the oxygen supply, carrying nutrients to the cells.
● It speeds up cell division and improves the synthesis of collagen, thickening the dermis and protecting against degenerative changes.

Controlling stress
If you are tense and anxious, this is often reflected in the condition of your skin. It may be paler than usual, be prone to spots, eczema or psoriasis and be susceptible to premature ageing.

Try to find what is causing your stress and aim to alleviate it as far as possible (see page 32). If necessary seek professional advice about solving the problem.

Sleep
Scientists do not understand fully why lack of sleep should result in dull, coarse skin, fatigue lines and slack muscle tone. However, they do know that getting adequate sleep is definitely one of the best beauty treatments!

A healthy diet
A balanced, varied diet is not only delicious to eat, but it is also an excellent way to keep the effects of ageing at bay. Make sure that you get plenty of the following:
Vitamin A is essential for the growth and repair of certain skin tissues. Lack of it causes dryness, itching and loss of elasticity. It is found in foods such as carrots, spinach, watermelon, broccoli and apricots.
Vitamin C is needed for collagen production and for maintaining a healthy immune system. It is found in citrus fruits, blackcurrants, cabbage, papaya, strawberries, tomatoes and watercress.
Vitamin E is an antioxidant that neutralizes free radicals (highly reactive molecules that cause ageing). It occurs in foods such as almonds, hazelnuts and wheatgerm.
Essential fatty acids, such as linoleic acid, found in sunflower, safflower and sesame seeds and nuts, and gamma linoleic acid

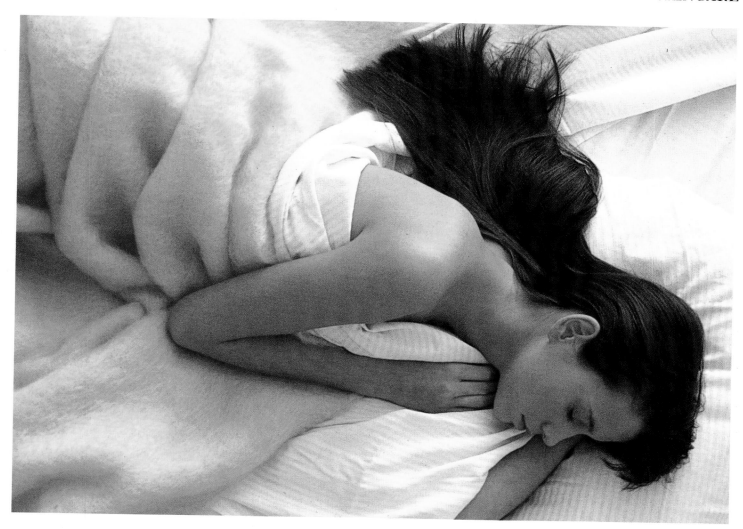

(GLA), found in evening primrose oil, prevent the skin from losing water and dehydrating.

Selenium is an antioxidant and protects against ageing.

Zinc works with vitamin A in the making of collagen and elastin.

Stop smoking!
The health hazards of smoking are, of course, reason enough to stop smoking, but the ageing effects on the skin are dramatic. Smoking causes lines around the mouth and eyes, drier, rougher skin and wrinkles as a result of pollutants in the smoke causing damage to the skin's collagen.

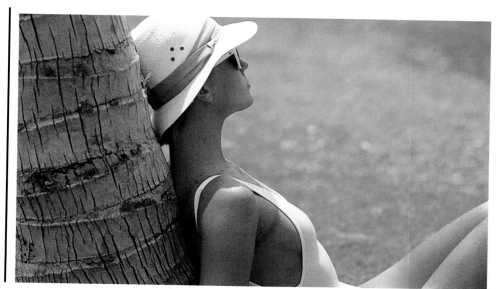

ENVIRONMENT

Protect your skin against adverse external conditions with action plans for every environmental situation.

In addition to changing with age, your skin can also change from day to day. The environment and the climatic conditions in which you live are major influences on the condition of your skin. Long-distance travel is a specially stressful situation for the skin. However, if you make simple adaptations to your skincare routine, you can stop problems *before* they start, avoiding the need for rescue operations that require time and effort.

DRY, HEATED ATMOSPHERES

Air-conditioning and central heating make life difficult for your skin. The humidity in some offices is lower than the Sahara Desert! As a result, the atmosphere robs your skin of precious moisture, leading to general dryness and flaking, and chapped – even cracked – lips.

Normal, dry and sensitive skins

These skin types suffer especially in dry atmospheres. The skin on your face may feel tight and you will be able to see fine lines on its surface. If this happens, use a slightly richer, creamier moisturizer.

Oily and combination skins

If your skin tends to be oily and you get spots, you may find that a hot indoor environment stimulates the sebaceous glands and makes the situation worse.

Use an oil-free moisturizer, blot any oil coming to the surface of the skin with a tissue and be sure to cleanse thoroughly night and morning.

Action plan for overcoming the effects of a dry, hot atmosphere

● Place bowls of water near radiators. The drier the room the faster the water will evaporate. Alternatively you could invest in a humidifier.
● Keep a check on the temperature indoors and, if possible, turn the thermostat down.
● Drink water throughout the day rather than tea or coffee. Remember that they are diuretics and cause water *loss*.
● Don't sleep in an over-heated room. This can cause fluid retention in the face, leaving you with a puffy complexion and bags under your eyes the next morning.

THE DEEP FREEZE

Cold, harsh weather conditions are the worst environmental challenge your skin will face.

Chilly temperatures restrict the blood circulation to the skin, so it looks pale and devitalized. They also make the texture of your skin rough to the touch and it often looks dull. The protective acid mantle is reduced too, as the glands are less active in cold weather. In addition, cold winds and dry atmospheres take moisture from your skin. After the age of thirty your skin's moisture levels naturally decrease, so it is even more vulnerable to adverse environmental conditions.

The effects cold weather have on your skin are as much as fourteen times worse when the air is also dry and can be ten times worse in high winds.

If you are skiing, your face is in for an even tougher time. At high altitudes, the lack of oxygen increases the skin's sensitivity to cold and the sun's ultraviolet rays dehydrate and age the skin.

Action plan for overcoming the effects of cold weather

● If you wash your face, do so at least half an hour before you go outdoors. This gives your skin a chance to dry thoroughly. If your face is slightly damp, the wind has an extra-drying effect.
● Wear a richer moisturizer.
● Wear night cream to replenish moisture lost from the skin during the day.
● If your skin is flaking, avoid *abrasive* scrubs. Use a very gentle exfoliator.

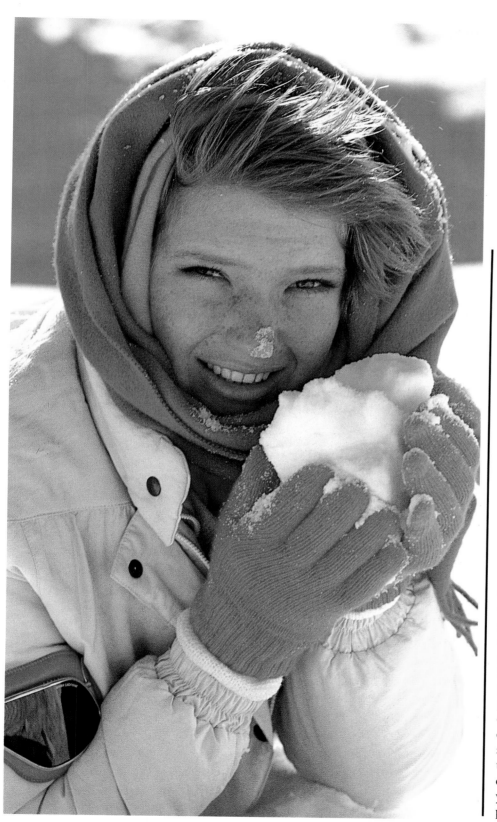

• Remember to care for your hands and nails, too, as the skin here can also suffer in cold weather.
• Always apply waxy lip salves or balms to your lips which are especially vulnerable to dehydration.
• Add moisturizing gels to your bath and apply body lotions every day to keep your skin soft.
• Never come in from icy cold weather and immediately roast yourself in front of a hot fire, as you will dry your skin excessively; the rapid contrast in temperature can also break capillaries, leading to red thread veins.
• If you are skiing or are outside in sunny, but cold weather, apply protective lotions on any exposed skin. In cold weather you will not be warned by the heat of the sun on your face that it may be burning. If there is snow it will reflect the sun, increasing its damaging effect. You will need special sun protection products if you are going to be out in sub-zero temperatures. Other products contain a higher percentage of water and may freeze on the skin, breaking the tiny capillaries. Use products specifically formulated to protect the skin in cold and windy conditions and use sunblocks on your lips. Reapply sun protection products frequently during the day.

HUMID HEAT

In humid, hot climates, cleansing is a top priority in order to remove oil and dirt, especially if you have oily or problem skin.

Action plan for overcoming the effects of humid heat

● Keep a mini skincare kit with you. Pack in it small or travel-sized bottles of wipe-off cleanser and toner and, if you need to, cleanse quickly at midday as well as morning and night, using tissues.
● Just use moisturizer where you need it and choose light or oil-free types rather than heavier creams.
● Wear a water-based foundation, especially if your skin is oily. If you prefer not to wear foundation during hot weather, just sweep on a little translucent or bronze powder to control any shine.
● Look out for oil-blotting lotions that can be worn under foundation to keep your skin matte and shine-free. Apply only over the T-zone.
● If you are working in a city, consider having facials more regularly to cleanse your skin of pollution residues. Your pores open up in hot weather and so absorb these residues more readily than when it is cooler.

HOT DRY WEATHER

Warm climates are not necessarily humid. When the weather is hot and dry, it is important to ensure that you protect your skin against moisture loss by wearing a moisturizer.

Apply a light, oil-free moisturizer where your skin tends to dry out easily and reapply it during the day if necessary.

TRAVELLING LIGHT

The air in planes is notoriously dry, leaving you feeling dehydrated and lethargic and your skin drained of energy and moisture. The tissues beneath the skin can become congested, too, and puff up, making you feel even more uncomfortable.

Action plan for overcoming the effects of flying

● As part of your final preparations before leaving, apply body lotion after you've showered or bathed. If you are travelling to a hot country and use self-tanning moisturizer, this will give your skin a colour boost for when you arrive.
● Carry a skincare kit in your hand luggage. As soon as you can, remove your make-up, freshen your skin with toner and spritz it with a mineral-water spray. Apply moisturizer and eye gel to ease any tendency to puffiness. If you are on a long-haul flight, repeat this routine when your skin feels dry, or use a moisturizer with extended moisturizing power – some moisturize the skin for up to twenty-four hours.
● Drink plenty of water and fruit juice to prevent dehydration.
● Avoid alcohol, tea, coffee and cola drinks as these actually have a diuretic effect.
● Move around as much as you can to stimulate your circulation.

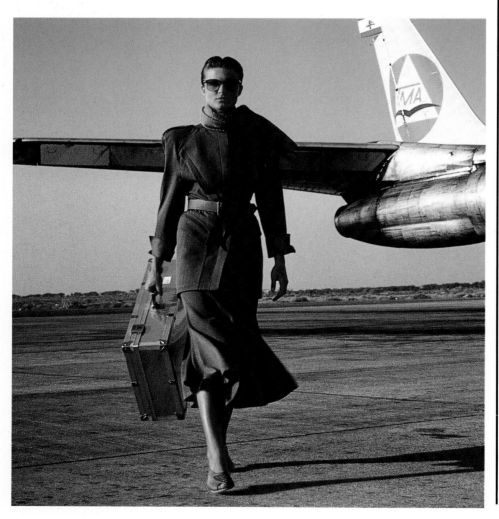

SPORTING CHANCE

You should cleanse your skin before and after you exercise and make sure that your sports kit and hair are as clean – and bacteria-free – as possible since they come into contact with your skin. Loose-fitting sports clothes in natural fibres are also kind to your skin. Do not wear a heavy moisturizer when exercising.

If you are going to be exercising outside, protect your skin by wearing a sunscreen. You can buy oil-free screens – gels for instance – which are terrific for oily skins. Apply sunblocks to vulnerable areas, such as lips, particularly if you are going sailing or windsurfing. Wearing sunglasses designed for your sport is also a good idea as they will protect your eyes and the skin around them from ultraviolet light and glare.

Always take a shower immediately after you've been swimming, so that the salt or chlorine in the water cannot dry on your skin and irritate it. When you are playing an active game, such as tennis or volleyball, pat perspiration from your face and body with a clean towel between sets and drink a refreshing glass of chilled water.

If you use the sauna or steam room at a health club, try not to stay in too long. Steaming in moderate amounts is good for your skin, but if you stay in too long the skin becomes dehydrated. Leave the steam room if your skin starts to turn red. Two to three minutes is usually plenty. Do not stay in more than about ten minutes, whatever your skin type. It is advisable to protect the delicate skin on your lips and eyelids with eye cream. Do not use a sauna or steam room if you have generally sensitive skin or broken capillaries.

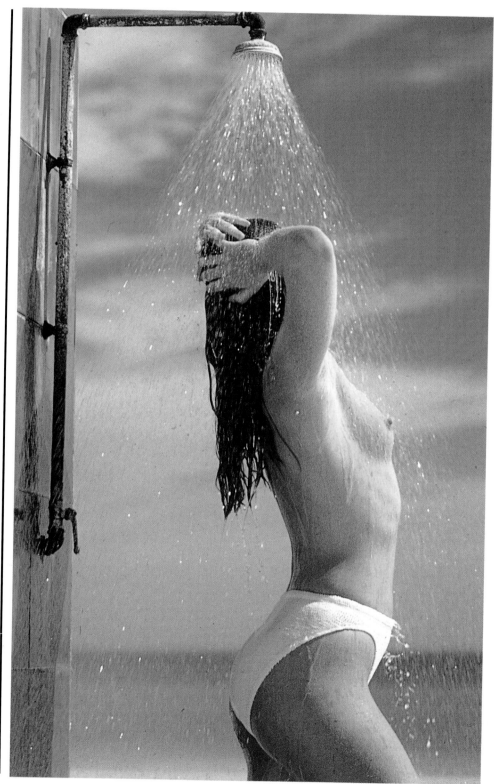

SUN AND TANNING

The key to the safest tanning is high protection with gradual exposure.

A tan makes us feel and look good. While dermatologists warn us of the dangers of sunbathing, there is a bright side to the sun. The sun's rays enhance our feelings of well-being – we feel relaxed and revitalized. They help our bodies to synthesize vitamin D which improves the absorption of minerals. There is also evidence that the full-spectrum light we receive from the sun reaches the brain via the eyes, stimulating the production of hormones, making us feel more energetic and improving our mood. Past research has shown sunlight to improve health problems such as respiratory infections, infertility, diabetes and stress-related complaints.

We now know, though, that if we are not careful we can pay a heavy price for a golden tan. The sun's ultraviolet rays damage the skin, breaking down the underlying supportive tissues and promoting wrinkles. Dermatologists believe that over ninety per cent of wrinkles are caused by sunbathing. Dehydrated, thinning, prematurely lined and blotchy skin is the cumulative result of sunbathing.

Sunbathing also increases the risk of developing skin cancer. The high numbers of new skin cancer cases reported in countries such as South Africa, Australia, New Zealand and the United States of America are the result of prolonged and intensive ultraviolet radiation on the fair skins of people of Celtic origin. However, even those people who sunbathe just once or twice a year on holiday are also at special risk. Studies have shown that the most dangerous form of skin cancer, malignant melanoma, can be caused by exposing skin that is unaccustomed to sunlight to a concentrated dose of ultraviolet light. Dermatologists now believe that a sun protection factor of at least 4 should be worn all year – even in countries such as Britain – beginning at birth, and throughout childhood and adulthood, particularly for outdoor leisure activities. It is a sore fact that just one sunburn in childhood can greatly increase the chances of developing a form of skin cancer.

Early detection of skin cancer is crucial if it is to be cured. If you notice any changes in the size or shape of moles on your skin, you should be seen by a specialist. Common sites for skin cancer include the side and nape of the neck, the eyelids, cheekbones (because of the reflection of sunlight on to them from the frames of your sunglasses), ears, lips (which contain no protective melanin) hands, legs and feet.

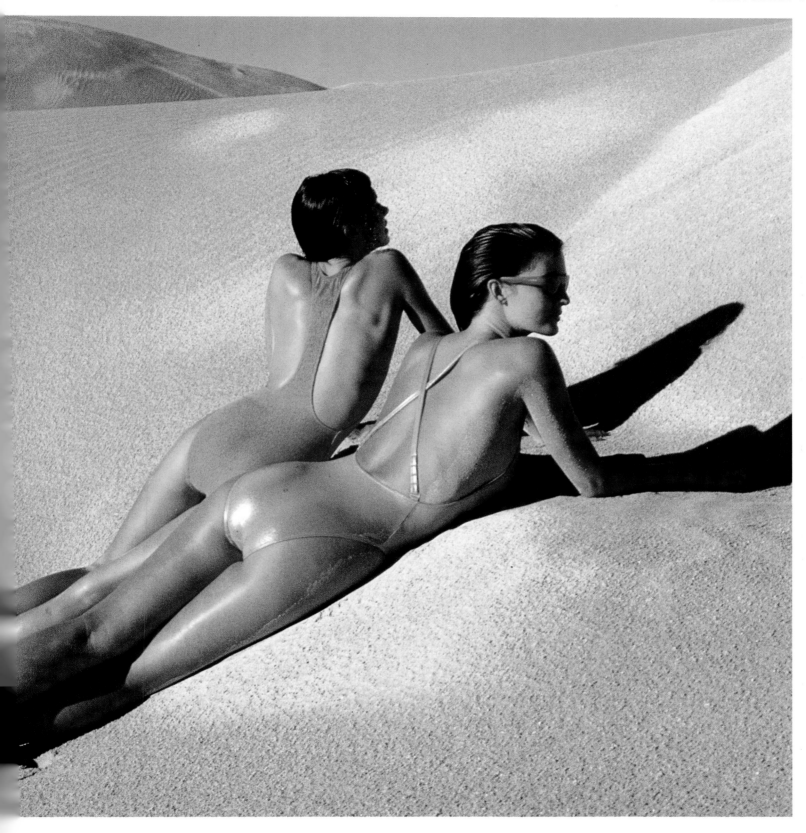

PROTECTION: THE SHORT CUT TO STAYING YOUNG

The good news is that protecting your skin from the sun and tanning *gradually* will cut the cost of sunbathing. You will develop fewer lines and greatly reduce the chances of suffering skin disease.

The key to safer tanning is to know your skin type and to use adequate protection.

Time your exposure to the sun

Your skin has built-in natural protection against the sun. The skin's pigment – melanin – will prevent your skin from burning for a short time if you are not wearing protection. This protection time ranges from ten minutes for very fair skins, which have very little melanin, to many hours for black skins, which contain a lot of melanin. If you multiply this natural protection time by the factor number of your sunscreen cream, you can work out how long you can sunbathe before you start to burn when wearing the sunscreen. The sunscreens recommended below should be used for at least the first two to three days while the skin steps up its production of melanin and you tan.

After this time, you can use a sunscreen with a lower factor, for example from SPF15 to SPF12, if your skin is not red or tender. Use this lower protection sunscreen for a few days and then step down to a lower factor again.

Sun protection tips if you are red-haired and freckled with pale eyes

This skin type always burns extremely easily and never tans.

Your skin's natural protection time is just ten minutes, so the recommended sunscreen for you is an SPF15 or higher. Use it throughout your holiday.

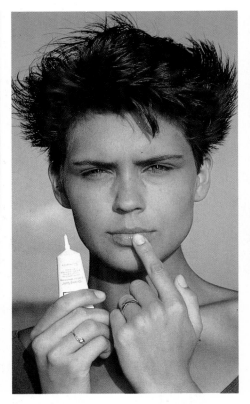

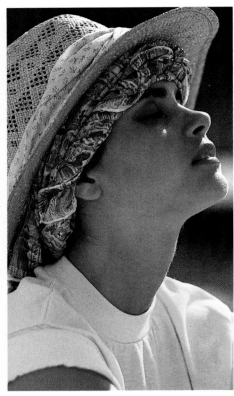

Fair skinned and blue-eyed

This skin type burns easily and tans minimally.

Your skin's natural protection time is ten to fifteen minutes. The recommended sunscreen for your skin is an SPF15 or higher.

Dark hair and eyes and pale skin

This skin type can burn and tans gradually.

Your skin's natural protection time is twenty minutes. A sunscreen of SPF10 or higher is recommended for you.

Olive skin and dark eyes

This skin type hardly burns at all and always tans, but still needs to be protected.

Your skin's natural protection time is between twenty and thirty minutes. The recommended sunscreen for your skin is an SPF6 to SPF8 or higher.

Dark olive skin

This skin type rarely burns and generally tans well.

Your skin's natural protection time is many hours. A sunscreen of SPF4 or higher is recommended.

Black skin

This skin type rarely burns and is deeply pigmented.

Your skin's natural protection time is many hours. A sunscreen of an SPF2 or higher is recommended for you.

TAKE EXTRA CARE

In addition to taking into account your skin's natural protection time when you sunbathe, you should also consider the following factors:

Time of day The sun's ultraviolet rays are most intense between eleven in the morning and three in the afternoon.

Temperature We gauge the strength of the sun by the warmth we feel, but the *infra-red* rays, which raise the temperature on the thermometer, are not a guide to the damaging potential of the *ultraviolet* radiation. Even on a cloudy day the ultraviolet rays are still quite powerful. Beware as well, when it is windy – the wind makes it seem cooler and we are lulled into a false sense of security.

Surroundings Sea, sand, snow and white buildings reflect light and can dramatically increase the effect of ultraviolet rays.

Latitude The sun is always overhead at the equator, giving your skin more concentrated doses of ultraviolet rays because they pass through less of the atmosphere before they reach you.

Altitude If you are taking a holiday in the mountains you're closer to the sun and the atmosphere is thinner, increasing the risk of sunburn.

All-round protection It is important to screen out both UVA and UVB rays. Not all sunscreens filter out both: choose one that does.

Extended protection The new sun preparations offer super-waterproof and long-lasting protection. Follow the directions on the product and re-apply it often if it is marked *water-resistant* rather than *waterproof*, if you are exercising (and therefore sweating your protection away) and after swimming. Sun gels are a great choice. They are cooling to the skin and won't block the pores. Remember that the sun protection factor that is right for your partner's or friends' skins is not necessarily adequate for yours.

Lips and eyes These need special care: avoid using normal sunscreens in the eye area. Wear high quality sun-glasses to prevent you from squinting and frowning and to protect your eyes from glare. Wear sunblock on your lips.

Sunscreens and skin repair

There is an added advantage to using sunscreens. Studies have shown that, if the skin is protected in this way, it can actually repair the damage done during previous periods of exposure to the sun. New collagen is formed and laid down on top of the damaged, cross-linked connective tissue.

After-sun skincare

● Remember to shower off salt or chlorinated water before it has time to dry on your skin and cause irritation.
● Use shower gels after sunbathing rather than soap, which will further dry sun-damaged skin.
● Lavish after-sun lotion on your face and body. It will contain skin-soothing and cooling ingredients, such as aloe vera.

Sunbeds

Using a sunbed may increase your skin's natural protection capacity. However, dermatologists strongly advise against using them. The risks of damaging your skin are high and one-third of the people who use them don't get a tan at all.

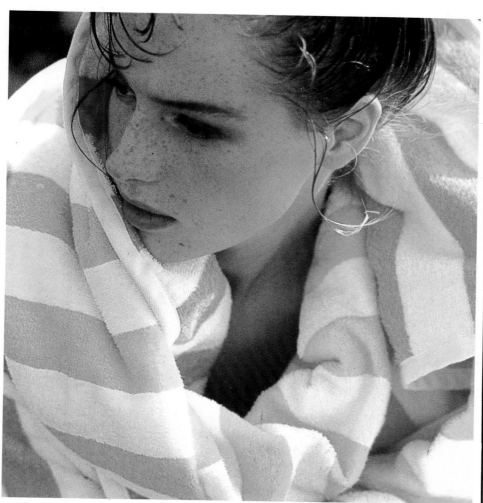

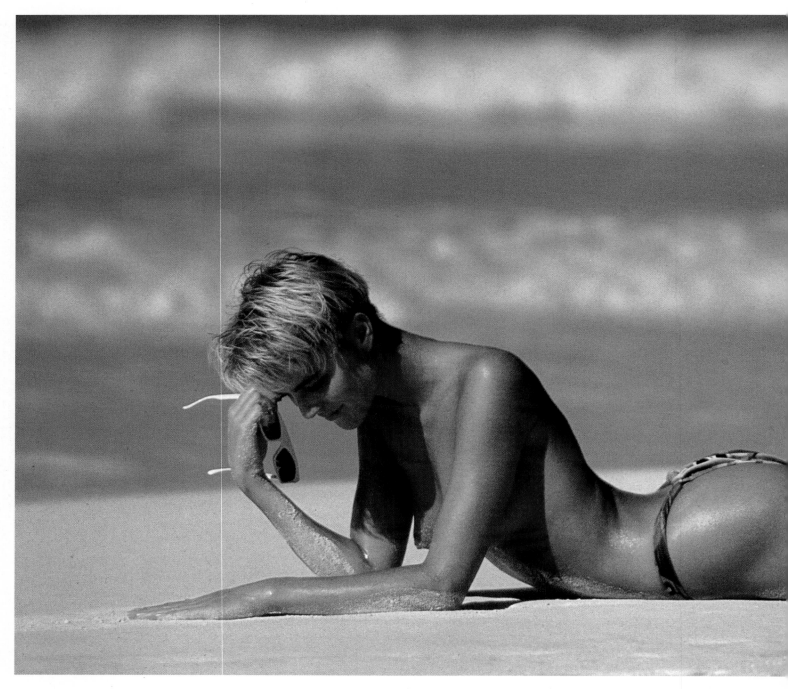

SHORT CUTS TO SOLVING SUN PROBLEMS

Sunburn
Sunburn has long-term detrimental effects on the skin and should be avoided. If you do burn, however, keep your skin cool and clean and soothe it with calamine lotion or natural yogurt.

If you burn badly over most of your body, you may need to rest in bed and drink plenty of fluids. You definitely should not sunbathe the

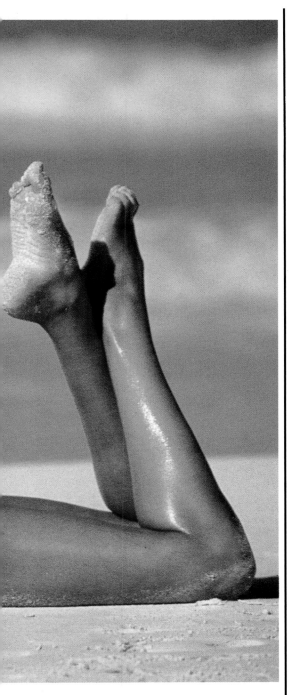

appearing on the chest, back and arms, and you can take steps to prevent it.

Avoid strong sunlight, especially between eleven in the morning and three in the afternoon when the sun is at its strongest. Wear high-factor sunscreens that screen out both UVA and UVB rays. Take cool showers or bathe frequently, patting the skin dry afterwards. Also avoid activities that make you sweat a lot.

If you do develop prickly heat, stay in the cool, apply calamine lotion or talcum powder and wear loose clothing.

Heat exhaustion and heat-stroke
Avoid succumbing to either heat exhaustion or heat-stroke by resisting the temptation to lie in the hot sun for hours on end. Keep your body cool by going for a swim at regular intervals.

Don't fall asleep in the sun. If you begin to feel woozy or headachey, retreat to the shade immediately and cool yourself down with cold compresses or a tepid bath and sip liquids. Orange juice is good because it replaces potassium lost through sweating.

Drink at least two litres (three to four pints) of water a day, and don't rely on thirst as an indicator of dehydration – you could easily be dehydrated and yet not feel thirsty. Don't drink alcohol or caffeinated drinks as these have a diuretic effect, adding to dehydration.

If, despite these precautions, you develop symptoms of heat exhaustion or heat-stroke, take the following steps immediately:
Heat exhaustion There are three types of heat exhaustion, all of which can be fatal: water deficiency, salt deficiency and anhidrotic.

The symptoms of water deficiency heat exhaustion include thirst, lack of appetite, giddiness, a dry mouth and rising temperature. Rest in cool surroundings and drink half a litre (about a pint) of water every fifteen minutes for two hours.

Seek medical help if your symptoms continue.

Salt deficiency heat exhaustion occurs if you have been sweating heavily during the first few days of acclimatization to a very hot climate and have not eaten properly. Fatigue, giddiness and severe muscle cramps are symptoms of this type of heat exhaustion. If you think you may be suffering from this condition see a doctor.

Anhidrotic heat exhaustion is a rare malfunction of the sweat glands, which occurs in people who have been in a hot climate for several months.
Heat-stroke The symptoms of heat-stroke are that your body temperature rises and you do not sweat, as this heat-regulating mechanism is not functioning correctly, you develop a severe headache, feel faint or disorientated, stagger or start to convulse. The skin is hot and may feel dry. 'Sunstroke' is an incorrect term – you can get heat-stroke without being in the sun.

Heat-stroke can be extremely dangerous, or even fatal, so call an ambulance or ask someone to drive you to the emergency department of a nearby hospital.

It is vital to cool a sufferer down by removing clothing and laying damp towels over body, hands and forehead. Keep fanning and spraying with cool water.

Photosensitization
The skin can react to plant and fruit juices, drugs or chemicals when you are in the sun, resulting in a sore, itchy red rash or blisters.

If you are going to sunbathe, avoid using perfume, aftershave, anti-bacterial soaps, artificial sweeteners, medications containing diuretics or tranquillizers.

Photosensitization can occur even if you have already been exposed to sunlight for some time.

Soothe the skin with cold compresses, showers and calamine lotion. Keep out of the sun.

following day, or until the redness has gone. Seek medical advice for severe burns.

Prickly heat
This spotty rash occurs as a result of blocked sweat glands, mostly

YOUR SKIN PROBLEMS SOLVED

There's no need to suffer in silence. Here are the solutions to some of the most common skin problems.

Q *I have small red veins around my nose. What treatments are available?*

A Thread veins are dilated capillaries that may have ruptured. They can occur at any age and affect any skin type, not just dry and sensitive skins. They occur most frequently on the cheeks, the bridge and sides of the nose, under the eyes and on the legs.

They are caused by sun damage, alcohol, drinking very hot drinks such as tea or coffee, eating spicy foods, high blood pressure, exposure to harsh weather conditions and steroid products applied to the skin.

You can disguise the veins using a concealer stick or you can go to a beauty salon where they will remove them by using either electrolysis or schlerotherapy.

With electrolysis a fine needle, which transmits shortwave electrical current, is used to cauterize the blood vessel, blocking off the flow of blood. Two or three sessions may be needed, depending on how many veins need to be removed. The skin swells for a couple of days and scabs may form at the point where the needle was inserted.

Schlerotherapy is used to treat more severe broken veins, particularly leg veins (but not varicose veins). A chemical is injected into the vein that makes it collapse and close up, the blood drying out and fading away.

Q *Can I avoid getting spots and what are the quickest ways to heal them?*

A The precise cause of acne is not known, although hormones play a key role in the appearance of spots. Acne often starts in teenage years because of this, and can last into the thirties, or longer. It can also flare up in women of thirty or even forty plus who have never previously suffered, because of a change in hormonal activity.

There are circumstances that can aggravate inflammation of the skin in some people:
● a very humid atmosphere
● certain medicines
● insufficient sleep
● pre-menstrual hormone fluctuation
● stress and emotional upsets
● the contraceptive pill
● the link with diet has not been proven, although an unbalanced diet and zinc deficiency may contribute
● certain ingredients in cosmetics may be a factor.

If you develop blackheads or acne, follow these precautions:
● Don't use harsh cleansing products or abrasive scrubs as this may increase the skin's oil production and will also dry the surface of the skin.
● Never pick at or squeeze spots – this pushes inflammation deeper into the skin and causes permanent damage.
● Salon facials and professional removal of blackheads are beneficial.
● Using clay masks at home absorbs excess oil.
● Contact your doctor if the problem is severe, but if you just have the odd spot, the best advice is to leave well alone and don't worry!

Q *Are fade creams safe to use to lighten pigmentation marks and darker skins?*

A Fade creams work, not by bleaching the skin, but by preventing the melanocytes in your skin from producing melanin, the skin's pigment. The results are not immediate, taking six or more weeks to have an effect.

The products sold in major chemists are considered safe when used correctly and are effective in 'lightening' pigmentation marks sparked off by a combination of the contraceptive pill and the sun, for instance. Look for fade creams with sunscreens if you're going to be spending time outside, and don't risk buying imported products from small shops if these contain more than the legal two per cent of hydroquinone or hydroquinone derivatives, as these can cause patchy pigmentation.

Q *How can I avoid stretch marks and are there any ways to remove them?*

A Stretch marks are caused by rapid fluctuations in weight, through dieting or as a result of weight gain during pregnancy, for example.

There is almost nothing you can do to avoid them in pregnancy as much depends on your hormones, although controlling your weight gain will help. Keeping your skin firm and elastic with body lotions can also be helpful. In addition, vitamins and minerals in your diet have been shown to maintain strong connective tissue.

Unfortunately, once the stretch marks have formed, no treatment or cosmetic will remove the scars. However, they will fade, even if they do not disappear completely, with time.

Q *How can I prevent cold sores occuring?*

A Cold sores are the result of a virus known as the herpes simplex virus 1. Once you have the virus it stays with you for life, although some people never have more than one outbreak. It can be activated by strong sunlight, colds and menstruation. Cold sores are extremely contagious and you must keep them clean and dry. Do not touch them or pass them to others through contact such as kissing.

Q *Can I have cosmetic surgery to remove frown lines and vertical lines on my upper lip?*

A No form of cosmetic surgery should be undertaken lightly. Always consult your doctor in the first instance, and, even if your doctor is unsympathetic, do not go to clinics that advertise. Remember that cosmetic surgery is painful and carries risks.

Cosmetic surgeons use collagen to fill out facial lines, some scars and wrinkles. Animal collagen is injected at intervals along the line. The effects last from six months to a year and need topping up as the collagen is absorbed by the body. It is not a treatment to be used by women or men in their fifties or later, as the skin will already have lost its elasticity. Allergic reactions are possible and tests must be carried out beforehand.

Q *How can I conceal dark circles under my eyes?*

A Dark circles are a very common complaint and can worsen with time as the surface skin thins. Try to get adequate sleep and on waking, tap the skin lightly with the fingertips, using a refreshing gel – this will improve circulation. Use a fine film of concealer, blending carefully.

Q *Could the flaking, red patches that have developed on my skin be psoriasis?*

A It sounds very likely. Psoriasis, unlike eczema, does not itch. It affects most commonly the scalp, elbows, shoulders, lower back and knees. The rough, red patches flare up at random and may be triggered by stress, shock, fatigue and depression. Studies are being carried out to determine the precise cause of psoriasis, which occurs when the skin cells turn over too quickly. The condition is often hereditary.

Your doctor can prescribe tar products or treatment by a form of ultraviolet, depending on the extent of the problem. Some doctors may suggest corticosteroid products, but these should be avoided as they lead to thinning of the skin. Alternative therapies such as acupuncture, using herb and plant oils and homeopathy can sometimes prove useful, as can bathing in mineral salts.

Eczema can also be helped by acupuncture and homeopathy. There are several forms of eczema, some of which are triggered by allergic reactions to particular chemicals. Your doctor can arrange tests to identify the cause.

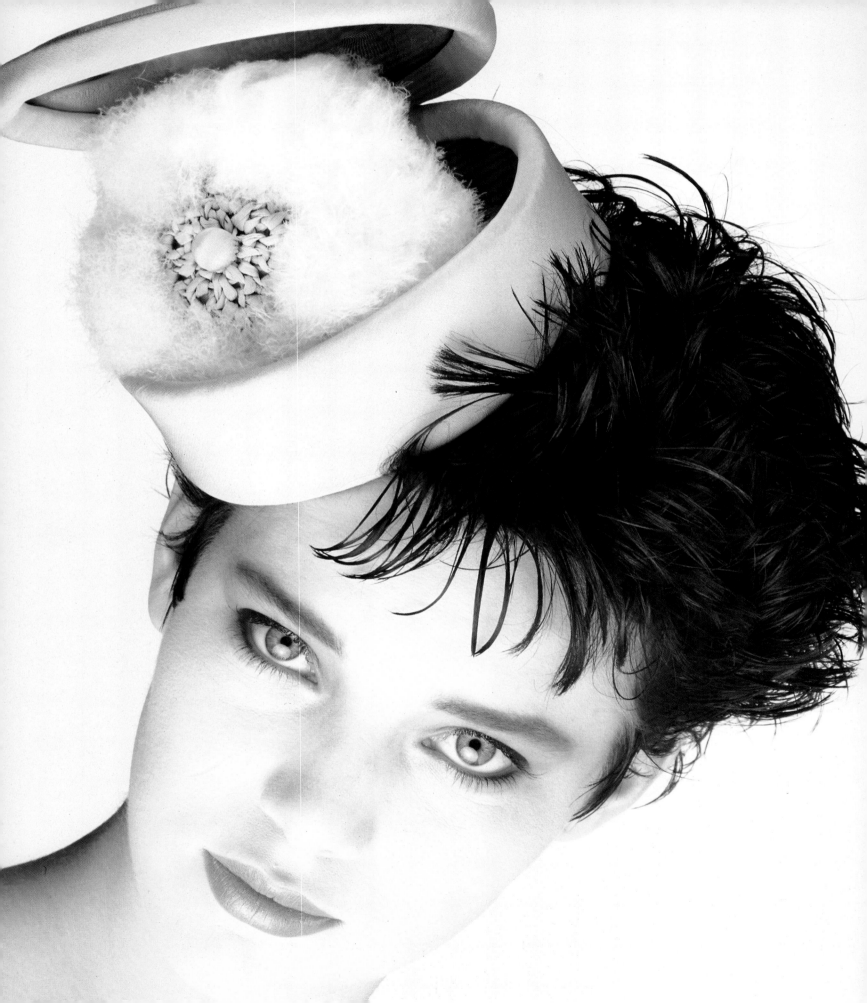

MASTERING MAKE-UP

Make-up is an art, but easy to master once you know the basics. In the following pages you will discover tips and tricks to help you maximize your looks fast, as well as plenty of inspirational ideas for creating looks for different occasions.

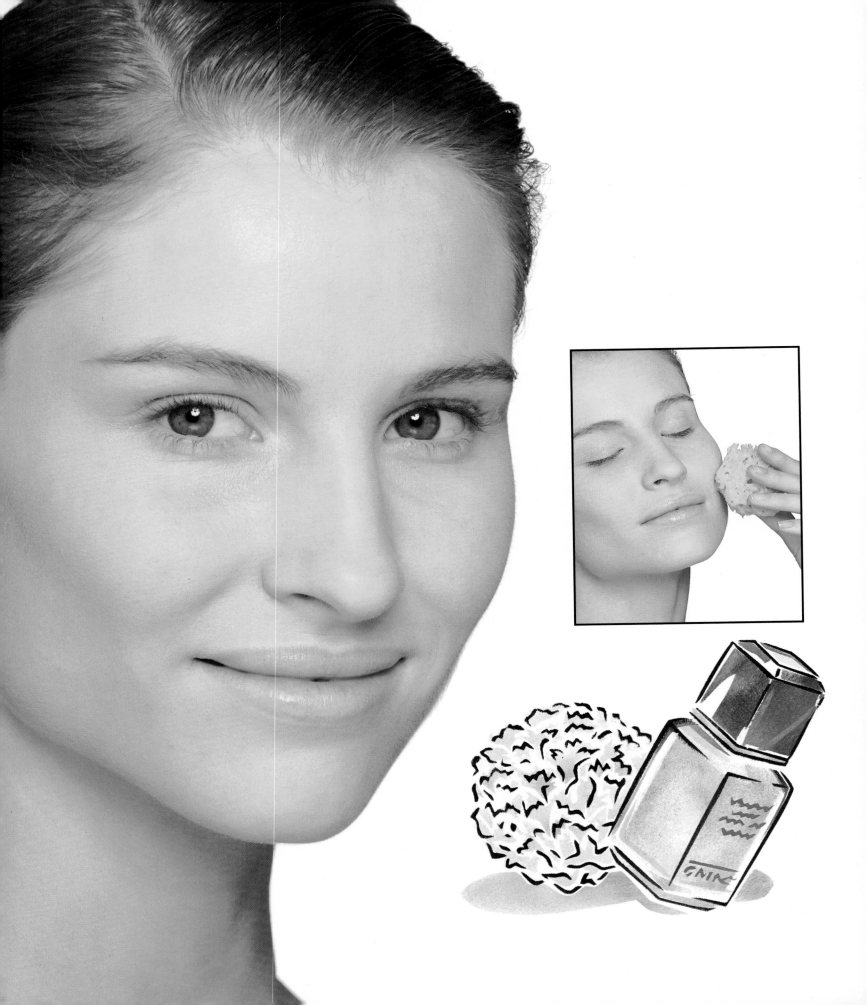

COMPLEXION PERFECTION

Carefully chosen products combined with professional techniques give you a flawless finish fast.

The key to successful make-up is getting the base right. This means choosing the right products for your skin type, learning colour and application techniques and having a knowledge of quick complexion enhancers for long-lasting polished perfection.

FOUNDATION

This has several beauty benefits: it evens out skin tones, smoothes the skin's texture, provides a base for your other make-up, keeping colours true, and protects your skin.

Choose a colour that is close to your own skin tone – going a few shades lighter or darker will look unnatural and mask-like.

Colour check

When buying a new foundation, choose the colour by applying a little on your jaw-line (don't use the back of your hand, as the skin here is darker and coarser than on your face). With a good match, the foundation will almost disappear. If you can't find an exact match buy a couple of foundations – one slightly darker, one slightly lighter than your skin tone – and blend them to your own ideal shade.

Tailoring foundation to your skin

Bear in mind your skin type and needs when buying your foundation.

It shouldn't look or feel uncomfortable. If it does, it is likely that you have chosen a product incompatible with your skin.

Remember the following when choosing foundation:
● If you have dry skin, look for a creamy, moisturizing formula.
● For oily or combination skin, an oil-free or water-based make-up is best as it minimizes shine (the high powder content in water-based foundations gives a matte finish).
● Hypo-allergenic bases are best if you have sensitive skin.
● Modern powder and cream mixes in compacts suit most skin types, except very dry skin. They are convenient and quick to use, are smoothed on with a sponge, like creamy foundation, and have a silky, powder-like finish.
● Tinted moisturizer does exactly what it says – leaves a tint on the skin and moisturizes. It is terrific for summer on tanned skin or for skin that is naturally clear and even toned, as it gives virtually no coverage; it doesn't work on open-pored or oily skin.

The coverage of a foundation depends on the density of the pigments it contains. As a general rule, the more solid a foundation is, the more coverage it will give.

Many foundations now also incorporate sunscreens to protect your skin from harmful ultraviolet light, which is an added benefit.

Application tips

For foundation to look like a second skin, you need to apply it correctly.

Always begin your make-up routine by cleansing and moisturizing your face. Whether you prefer to apply your make-up in daylight or artificial light, make sure there are no shadows. It may seem obvious, but if you make up in inadequate or unbalanced lighting, this will cost you precious time later as you try to retouch mistakes.

Dampen a make-up sponge and then squeeze it well in a towel so it is just slightly damp. A triangular wedge shape or a natural sponge is best for applying foundation – they cover more efficiently and blend better than fingers.

Using the back of your hand as a palette to mix from, dab dots of foundation on your forehead, cheeks, nose and chin. Work the sponge in quick, downward and outward movements, remembering to blend to just under the jaw-line to avoid any 'tide-marks', but don't take foundation down on to your neck. Fade the foundation out towards your hair-line, avoiding taking it into your hair.

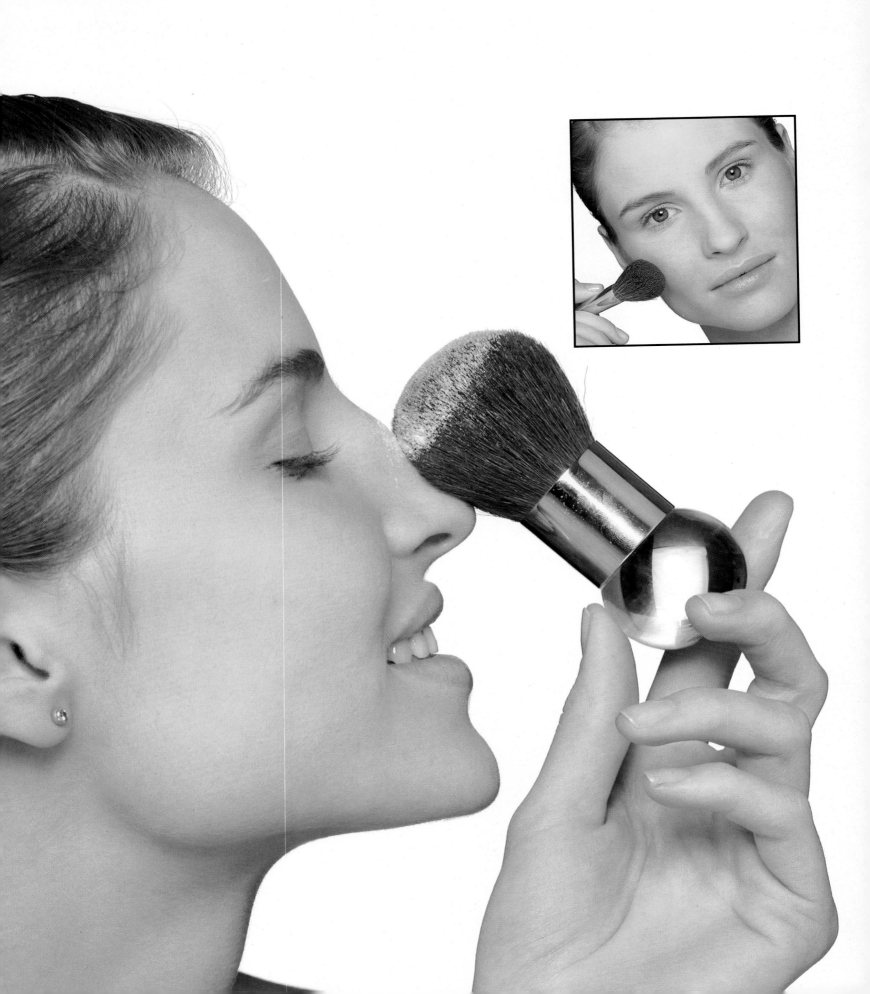

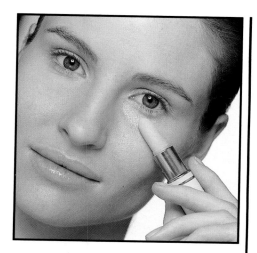

CLEVER CONCEALER

Concealers are fast, effective tools for disguising blemishes, shadows, scars and red veins.

Application tips

Pick a shade slightly lighter than your foundation and apply it *over* foundation. Sweep on lightly from the tube or dab some on your fingertip and press it on, using the barest minimum, then tidy up the edges with a flat, slim brush.

POWDER

Face powder, which went through a period of not being fashionable, is back as an indispensable beauty tool. Its traditional function is to 'set' make-up, giving it a finished look. However, modern, fine-textured powder can be a good base in itself, worn simply over moisturizer. This is a terrific time-saver when you are in a hurry or don't want to wear foundation, but don't want to be completely barefaced either.

Application tips

Loose powder should be applied with a large, soft brush (larger than your blusher brush) or pressed on with a velour pad in order to set make-up thoroughly. Brush off any excess with your powder brush.

Pressed powder is applied with a pad and is particularly suitable for retouching make-up during the day. For the most natural finish (matte and invisible) use a translucent powder. It reflects light to give the skin a luminous, satiny quality. Heavily pigmented powders are out-dated, usually look artificial and are generally best left well alone!

Colour correction powders are brush-on instant beautifiers. They come in pressed or loose form and are simply applied over foundation in the areas they are needed. Use them individually as follows:

White adds luminosity to the complexion and is particularly good for evening.

Mauve/violet warms up a sallow complexion.

Green tones down high colour.

Pink gives a healthy glow to pale skin.

Blue tones down high colour.

Apricot gives a healthy glow to olive skin that lacks brightness.

BLUSHER

The fastest face shaper, blusher adds a gentle bloom of colour to the cheeks and shape to the face.

On the whole, powder blusher is simpler and quicker to use than cream, but whichever you prefer, remember not to overdo it. It is, after all, intended to mimic the natural glow of your cheeks.

Choose a blusher colour that will co-ordinate with your total make-up look. Try to avoid the frosted variety – they can look attractive if you have a suntan but tend to be rather ageing otherwise.

Application tips

To apply powder blush, using a large, soft brush, start the colour on the 'apples', or fullest part of your cheeks, directly below the centre of your eyes.

Smile and dust the blusher over your cheek-bones, upwards and outwards. Fade the colour towards, but not into your hair-line.

Well applied, cream blusher can look very natural and fresh. Using the same sequence as described above, dab a couple of dots of colour on the apples of your cheeks and blend them well with either a damp sponge or fingertips, again using an upward and outward motion.

Quick blusher tips

● *If you find you have put on too much blusher, apply a light film of foundation – this will tone it down.*

● *Apply powder blusher over your foundation and powder. Apply cream blusher before your powder.*

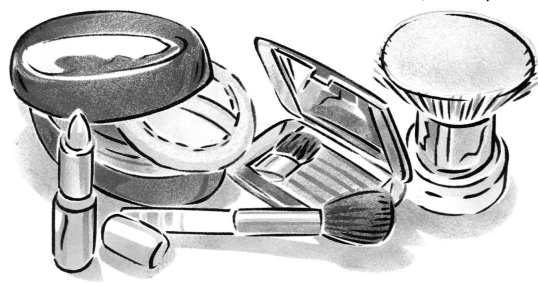

EYES RIGHT

Make the most of your eyes – choose colours that flatter and apply them so that they last .

We usually notice the eyes first when we look at someone. Whatever the colour and shape of your eyes, there are myriad ways to enhance their natural appeal.

EYESHADOW
Use eyeshadow to complement the colour of your eyes. If you wear a colour that matches them, you may detract from their beauty. As a general rule, if you have pale eyes, choose from browns, plums, pinks and purples. Colours that flatter dark eyes are greys, dark blues, burgundy shades and yellows.

When using more than one colour, it is best not to mix shades from different colour families: cool blue, for example, looks wrong with warm gold. A short cut to getting colour combinations right is to buy a palette containing two or more toning shades.

Clashing make-up colours can be fun, but they need to be applied flawlessly and your colouring must be able to take it. Orange and yellow eyeshadows with pink lipstick look great on some brunettes, but look too garish if you've got dyed blonde hair, for instance. It is best to keep colours subdued for day and bring out the brights for evening glamour.

Here are some tips to help you choose the right eyeshadow for the effect you want.

Pressed powder eyeshadows give excellent coverage and are useful for building up colour intensity; the colours also keep true during wear.

Loose eyeshadow powders tend to be pearly and slightly finer textured than pressed and are best used as highlighters or for a soft sheen on bare lids.

Cream eyeshadow is by far the most difficult to use and it tends to sink into the crease of the socket-line after a few hours.

Application tips
You will need to include two types of brush and an applicator in your make-up kit:
- a firm, flat brush for applying all types of shadow
- a sponge-tipped wand to place and build up colour
- a softer brush to blend colour.

Tap off any excess powder from your brush before applying it, so that you can make sure it goes where you want it to go. It is better to add more as necessary rather than have to rectify mistakes or even start the process all over again.

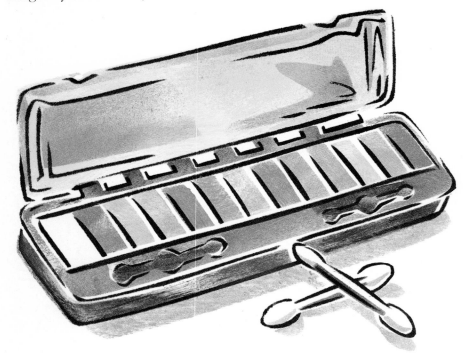

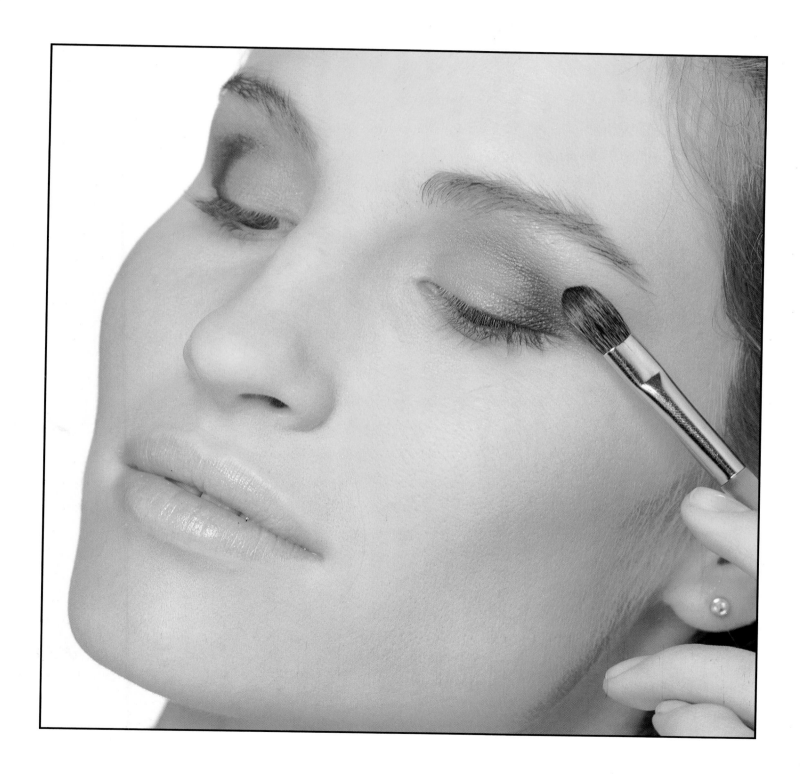

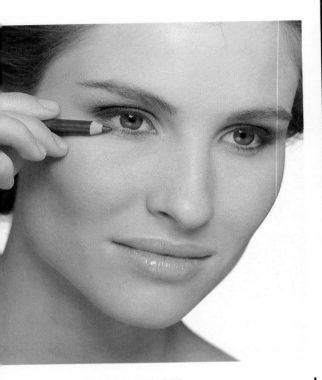

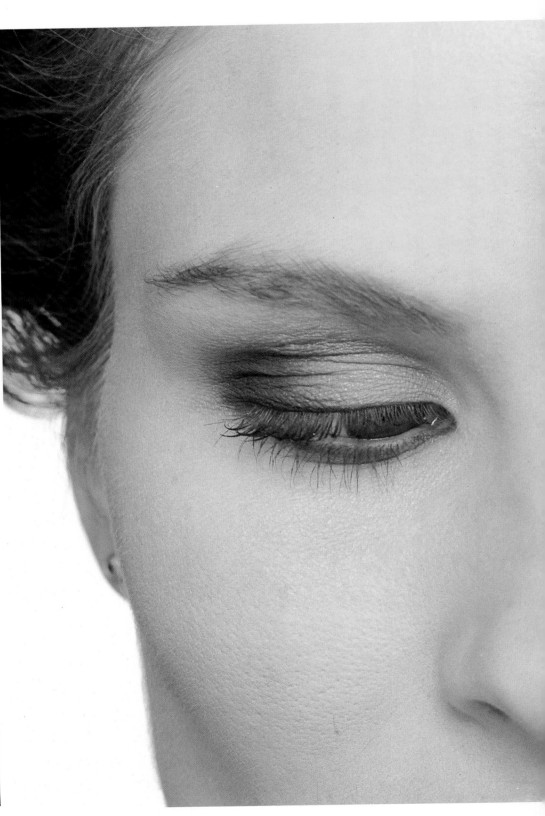

EYE-PENCIL
An eye-pencil gives instant emphasis to the eyes. It has most effect when you use it to draw a line close to your lashes (upper and/or lower) and then smudge the line with a soft brush. In fact, many eye-pencils come ready equipped with a smudger at one end.

Grey, brown or other softly coloured pencils are good for daytime, and, like eyeshadows, the more dramatic colours look great for evenings or sunny holidays.

EYELINER
Most eyeliners are fluid and you apply them with the brush provided in the cap. Well applied, liquid eyeliner gives a precise and very positive shape to the eye.

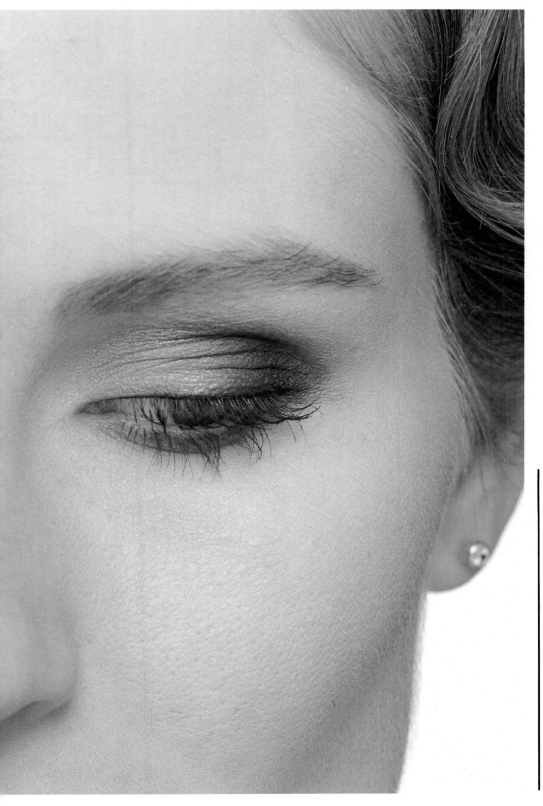

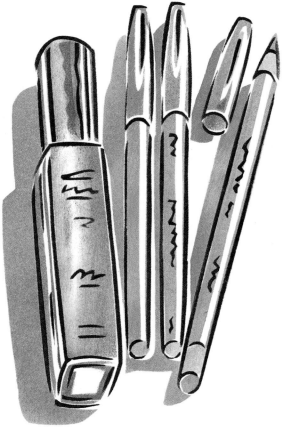

MASCARA

Normally two or three coats of mascara are ample. Comb through your lashes after the final coat so that they don't clump together.

Consider, too, having your eyelashes dyed at a salon. This looks very natural and, particularly for women with very fair lashes, saves time in your make-up routine.

Quick mascara tips

● *If your mascara is drying out, place it – sealed – on a radiator or into a beaker of warm water for a minute and you will get a couple of extra applications out of it.*

● *If you are in a rush, apply one coat of mascara to your upper lashes only. This will have the effect of instantly 'opening' your eyes.*

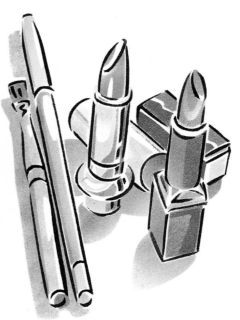

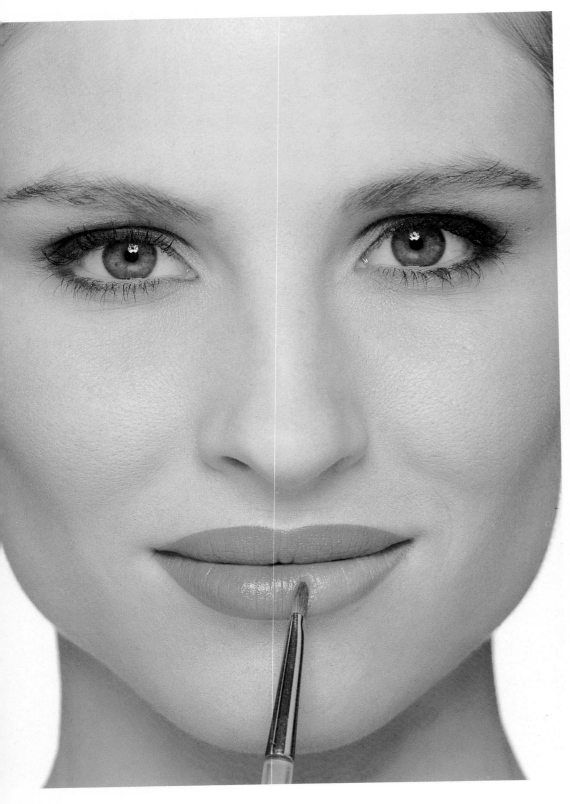

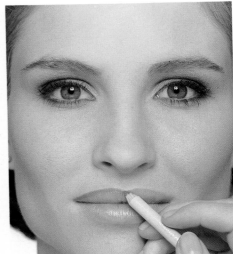

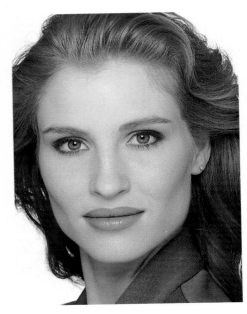

LIP SERVICE

Whether you choose palest pink or striking scarlet, here are the quickest lip tips for a perfect finish every time.

Research suggests that we choose a lip colour to reflect our moods – vibrant colours when we feel confident and want to be noticed, and paler shades when we feel introverted or even low.

Whether this is true or not, there is a cornucopia of products to colour and protect your lips – lipsticks, glosses, lip powders – many enhanced with moisturizers and ultraviolet filters. Whichever colour you choose, for whatever reason, remember these five tips:
● Before applying lip colour, prepare your lips with moisturizer or a specially designed lip primer, so that the colour goes on evenly and lasts longer without feathering.
● A lip brush gives a professional finish to your lips.
● It is not essential to use lip pencil (you can get a good finish with a primer and brush alone) but if you do want to use lip pencil, for instance with a very vibrant lipstick that needs a precise outline, it should be the *same* colour as the lipstick or slightly paler – a darker outline does not look attractive.
● Avoid frosted lipsticks as they rarely enhance your teeth or the shape of your mouth.
● Choose a lip colour to pull a look together, but, remember, as a general rule, blue-toned (rather than orange-toned) reds and pinks

and browns will make your teeth appear whiter.

Before going out in the evening or for a special highly polished finish it is worth taking time over applying your lipstick.

Application tips
Begin by priming your lips with moisturizer and/or lip primer. If you are using a lip pencil, draw in your lip outline very carefully. The pencil shouldn't drag at your mouth, so warm it up slightly in the palm of your hand first to soften it. Try resting your little finger on your chin for balance.

Load your lip brush with colour and brush inwards from the corners of your mouth. To give your lips the Cupid's bow shape, lie the brush flat to paint a 'V' shape or curve.

Blot your lips with a tissue, dab on a little face powder and repeat with a second layer of colour.

If time is very tight, choose lipsticks that give a fairly sheer layer of colour. They are quick to apply straight from the lipstick bullet and do not need outlining or blotting.

TERRIFIC TEETH
A beautiful smile depends on healthy teeth. To achieve this, regular care is essential and this means choosing a good toothbrush. A toothbrush that has a small head

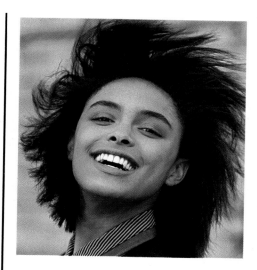

is best because it will reach all your teeth and gum margins. Check too, that your brush has medium bristles with rounded ends. Electric toothbrushes are super-efficient at cleaning teeth.

Use dental floss from time to time to clean between your teeth, but be gentle and careful so as not to damage your gums.

Cosmetic dentistry has made a great deal possible:
● New materials mean that laminate veneers bonded to individual teeth don't pick up stains or plaque and last many years.
● White fillings are now much more widely available, replacing the silver-coloured ones.

5-MINUTE MAKE-UP

Classic, neutral colours and simple techniques are the success for a super-quick make-up.

Here are the make-up tricks for those days when you haven't got a second to spare – in the morning, especially, when you're dashing to work, or running the children to school.

The secrets are to keep colours neutral and to choose products that give a featherweight finish. Plan your make-up colours around your clothes – and don't deviate to experiment with new ideas when every minute counts. Save them for the weekend.

● First, dab a little moisturizer on to clean skin or apply tinted moisturizer. If you wear foundation, pick the sheerest base you have and apply it with a damp make-up sponge. Remember to take the foundation over your lips too. If you apply your foundation with your fingertips, take a few moments to blend it using a slightly damp latex sponge.

● For eyes, use a flash of eye pencil on the upper and/or lower lid in brown, black, navy or grey, blended with your finger or with an eyeshadow applicator.

● Apply a little, pale matte eyeshadow up to your brows.

● Apply one coat of mascara, blot the brush on a tissue and then sweep it across your brows.

● Apply translucent face powder, brushing all over the face in every direction.

● Use powder blusher – it's quicker than cream blusher.

● Finally, pick a matte lipstick in a mid-shade (anything too dark takes too long to apply accurately). Forget lip pencil unless you're an expert at using it. You can't expect lipstick to last all day, so apply a fast coat from the tube and re-apply as necessary later.

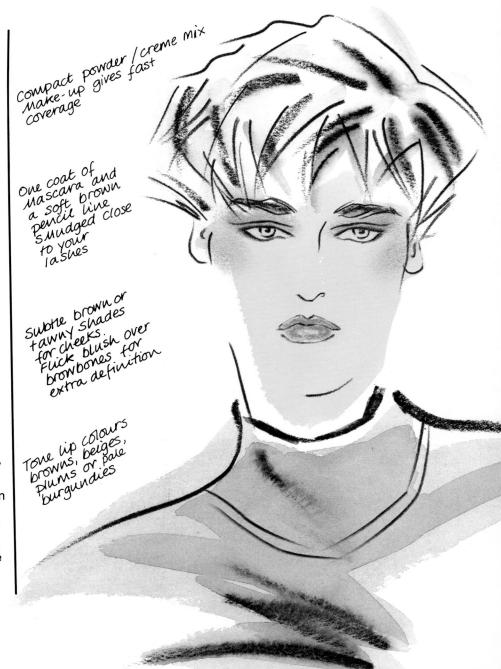

Compact powder /creme mix make-up gives fast coverage

One coat of mascara and a soft brown pencil line smudged close to your lashes

Subtle brown or tawny shades for cheeks. Flick blush over browbones for extra definition

Tone lip colours browns, beiges, plums or pale burgundies

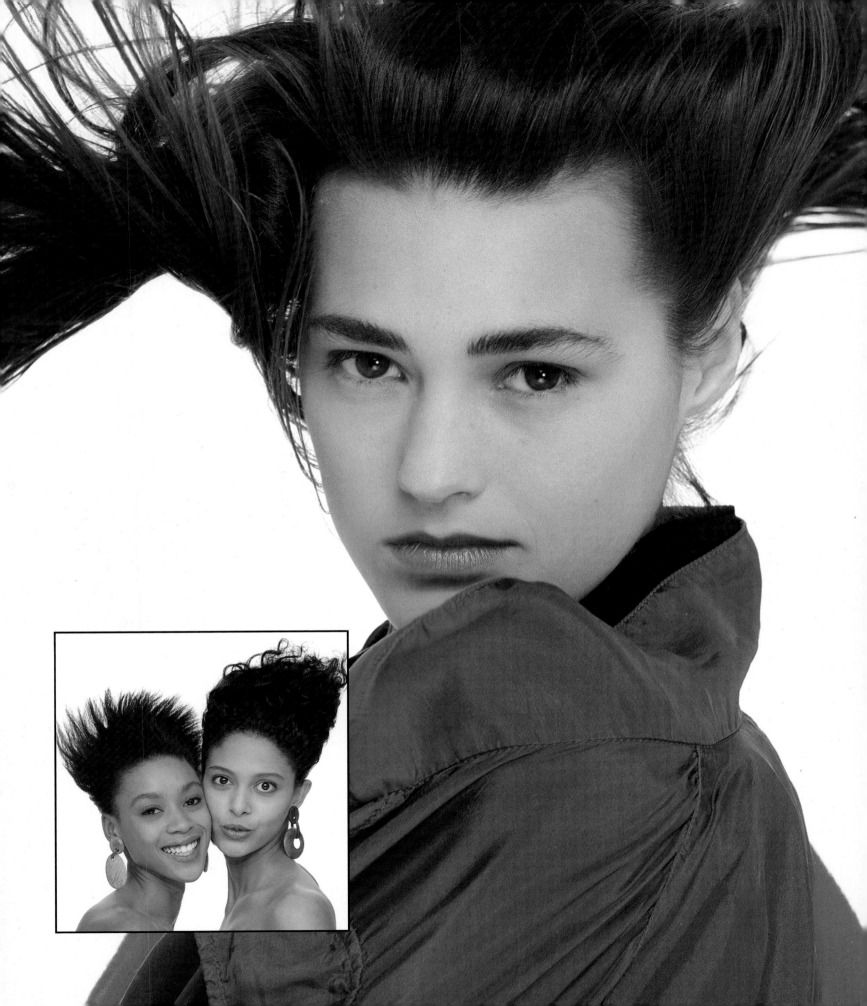

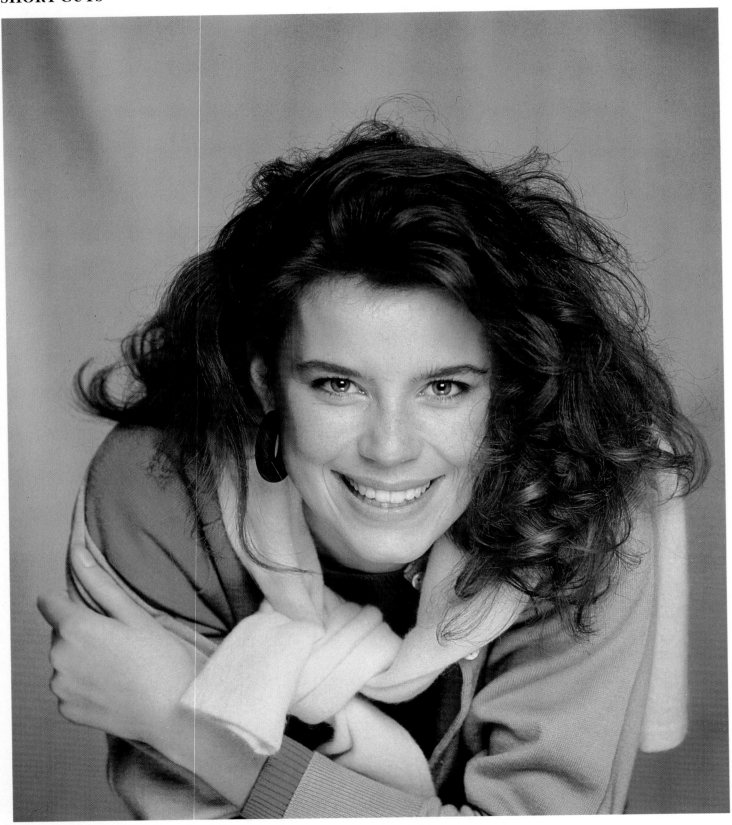

THE FRESH COUNTRY STYLE

If you're looking for the fresh glow that looks right in the open air, here's a step-by-step guide to the perfect shades.

The route to a glowing complexion and minimally made-up look is to keep your technique simple and to choose country colours.

Avoid heavy foundations when you're outside and skip face powder – it looks unnatural in bright sunlight. Don't try to hide freckles, they enhance the fresh-air feel of this style.

Tinted moisturizers are excellent for normal to dry skins. Many of them contain broad-spectrum ultra-violet filters and so offer a small degree of protection against the sun's ageing rays.

You may find that tinted moisturizers can accentuate the appearance of open pores on oily skins. If this is so in your case, try bronzing powders instead. Look for bronzers with only a tiny amount of shimmer for the most natural appearance.

For wide-awake eyes, shades of green work well for the outdoor life. Teal and hyacinth blue are also possibilities, but choose matte eyeshadows when applying a pastel shade. Cream shadows that are crease-resistant formulations are also worth trying.

Keep mascara to the minimum. Waterpoof mascara is useful for active days, but remember that you'll have to remove it with a specially-formulated lotion or gel. The clear mascaras which thicken lashes and give them a gloss are great for dark lashes, and can also be used to tame eyebrows.

Cream and gel blushers create a flushed-with-the-sun effect and look more natural than powder blushers. Using your fingers or a make-up sponge, apply just a little to moisturized skin and blend well.

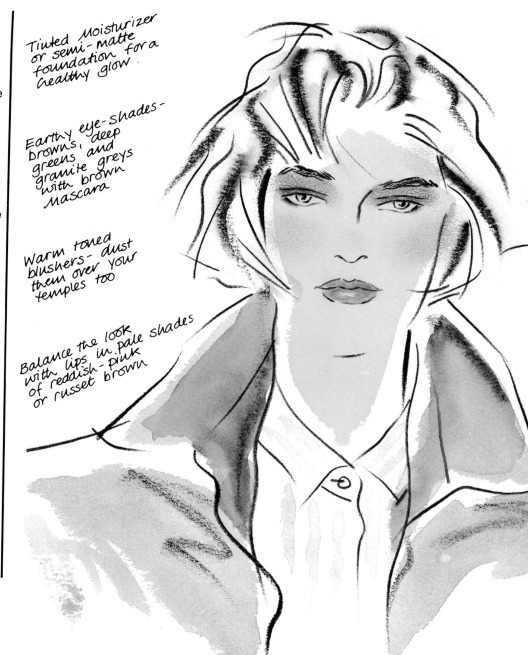

Tinted moisturizer or semi-matte foundation for a healthy glow

Earthy eye-shades – browns, deep greens and granite greys with brown mascara

Warm toned blushers – dust them over your temples too

Balance the look with lips in pale shades of reddish-pink or russet brown

THE CLASSIC FACE

Soft and beautifully balanced, the classic make-up uses face-flattering colours that flow together.

The perfect beauty of a classic make-up is easy to achieve if you follow a few ground rules. The essence of this timeless style is harmony: lips, cheeks and eyes are all beautifully balanced, with no single area stronger than the others. To achieve a classic look you should always bear in mind that you are creating a natural-looking make-up that subtly enhances your features.

Bright colours and fantasy looks are out of tune with the classic face. Instead, choose soft shades that are in tune with each other: for brunettes through to blondes, soft apricots on lips and cheeks work well with earthy browns on eyes; for blondes, pale pink looks pretty with navy blue. A certain winner when choosing eye colours is to complement tones in your natural hair colouring. Keep to one eyeshadow shade on eyes, or use two shades that are very similar or classic shades that are complementary.

The colours in this soft make-up style are always carefully blended. Smudge eye-defining lines and blusher slightly to avoid hard edges.

The classic woman wears more make-up than the all-natural, country fresh girl. Timeless elegance calls for a radiant complexion that tends towards the pale but radiant rose. Liquid foundation will give a porcelain complexion. Apply just enough to even out any imperfections.

Face powder completes the velvety finish. Apply powder after eye and blush colour, but before your lipstick, dusting it on very lightly and taking a few seconds to fluff off any excess.

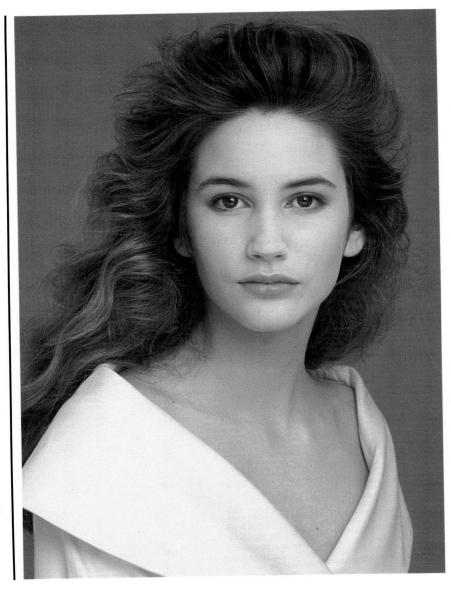

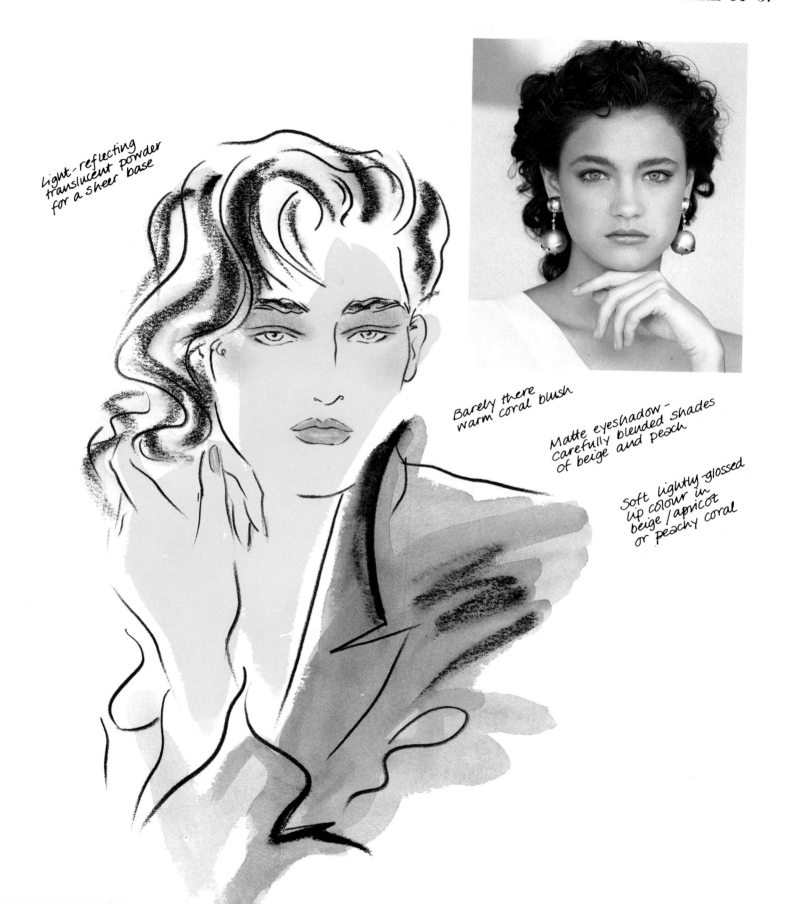

Light-reflecting translucent powder for a sheer base

Barely there warm coral blush

Matte eyeshadow – carefully blended shades of beige and peach

Soft lightly-glossed lip colour in beige/apricot or peachy coral

THE MODERN GRAPHIC LOOK

Self-assured and dynamic, the dramatic red-lipped, dark-eyed beauty uses colour to make an impact.

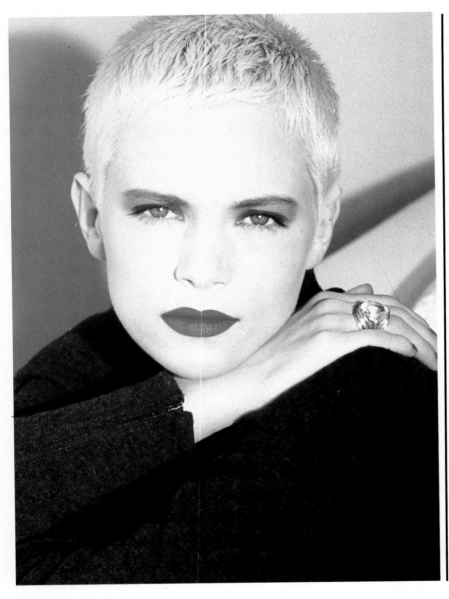

Monochromatic eyes set against a chalky white complexion and assertive red lips: this is a powerful, high-fashion image for the contemporary woman.

Foundation that is often paler than the natural complexion colour is applied to cover the skin well. Pressed powder, often with a slight lilac tint, is applied next to ensure the base stays matte and shine-free.

Black or steel-grey eyeliner is an essential component of the look. Draw a neat line along the top lid, starting at the inner corner of the eye where the line should be finer and increase the depth of the line from the centre of the eye to the outer corner. If you like, you can wear a matte eyeshadow from your lids up to your brows, or leave the eyes bare.

Eyebrows are either thick, straight and heavily pencilled-in or finer and very arched, 1940s style. Before you draw in your brows, brush them against the direction of the hair to remove excess powder, then brush them back again. Use a black eyebrow pencil to shape and shade the brows so that there is a solid line.

Matte lipstick in cardinal red or bordeaux is applied with a lipbrush to create a wide, full mouth. Choose a good quality, long lasting lipstick. By blotting your lips, applying powder, then another coat of lipstick and then blotting again to finish, the colour will stay strong and the line will not bleed or smudge.

It is generally best not to use blusher, which softens the effect, but if you prefer to wear some, try applying a light touch of colour at the very outer edge of the cheekbone.

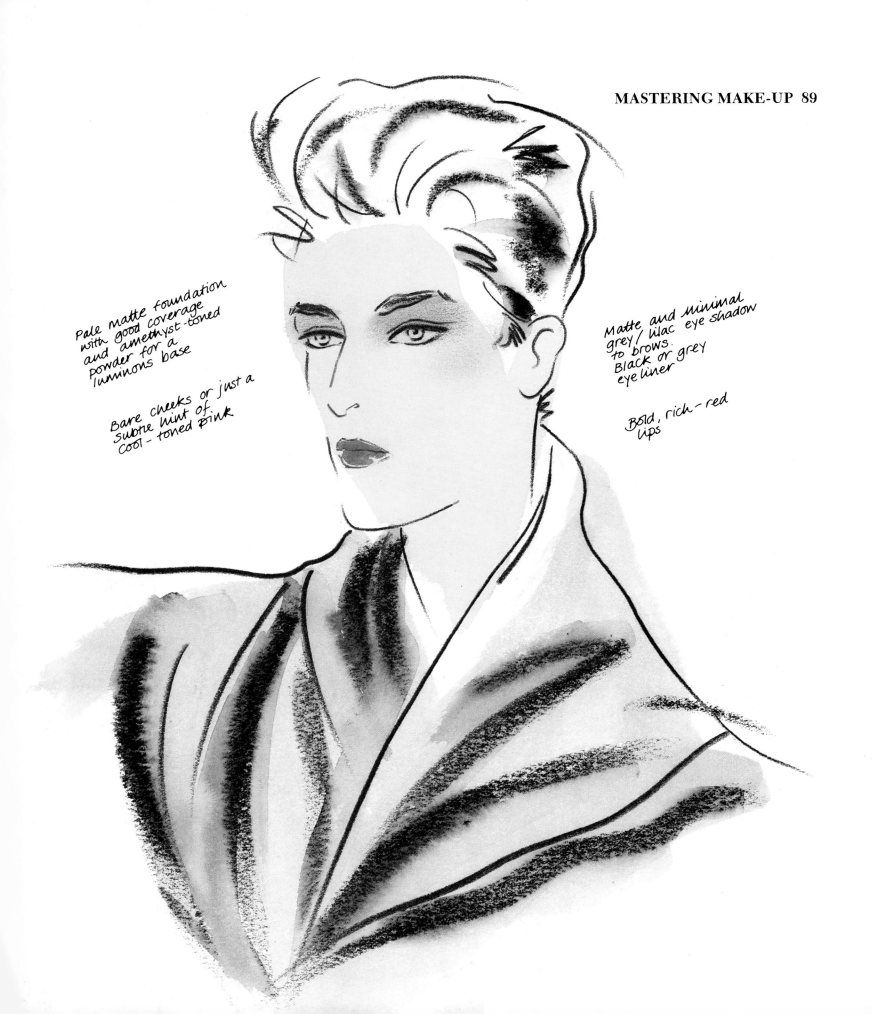

Pale matte foundation with good coverage and amethyst-toned powder for a luminous base

Bare cheeks or just a subtle hint of cool-toned pink

Matte and minimal grey/lilac eye shadow to brows. Black or grey eye liner

Bold, rich-red lips

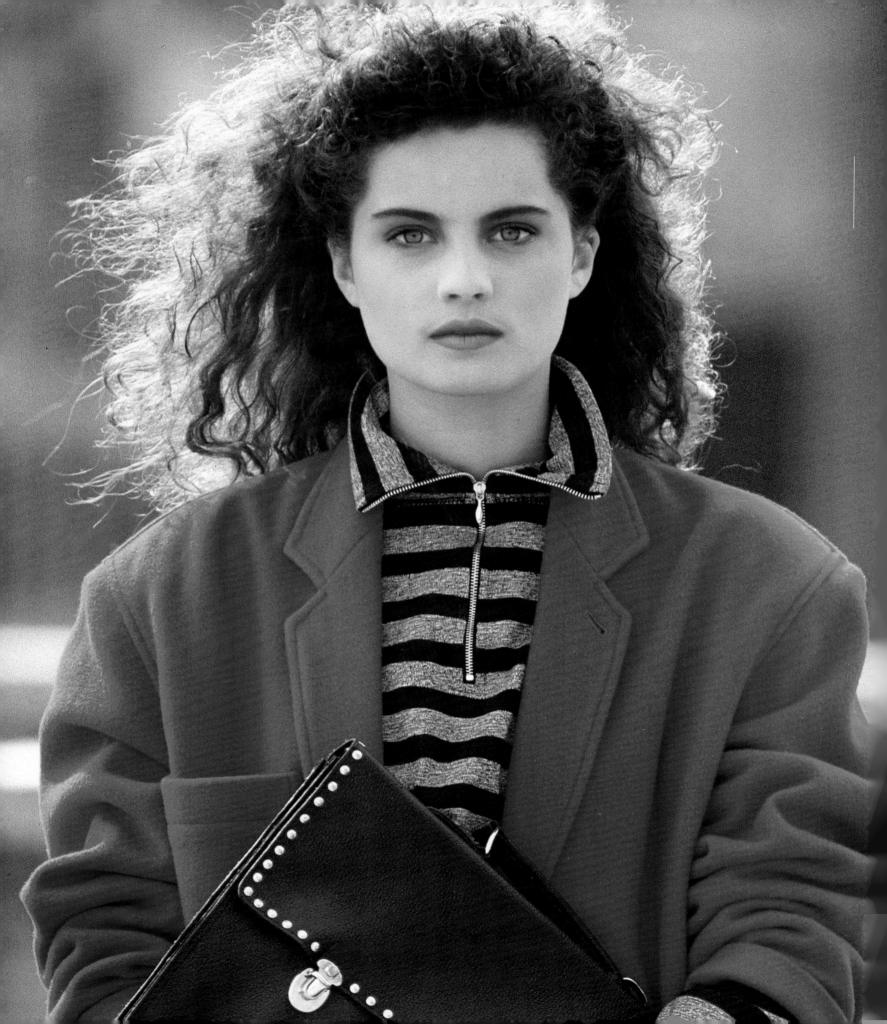

THE WORKING IMAGE

Make-up is an essential tool in creating a professional appearance.
Take our short cuts to a super-successful face.

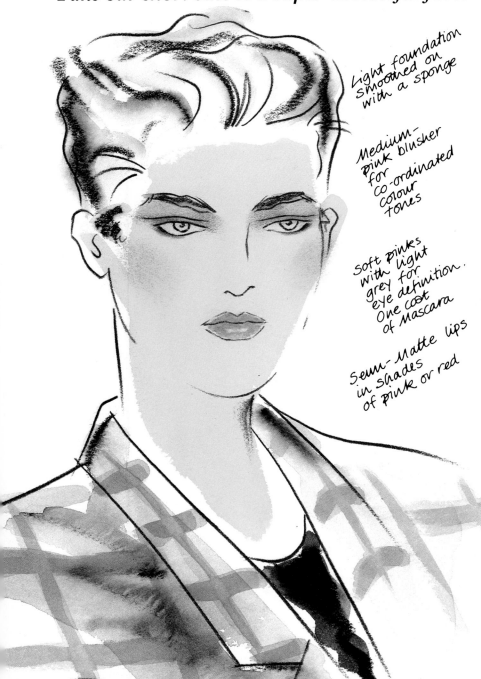

Light foundation smoothed on with a sponge

Medium-pink blusher for co-ordinated colour tones

Soft pinks with light grey for eye definition. One coat of Mascara

Semi-Matte lips in shades of pink or red

Make-up is an essential tool in putting together a successful working face. It makes us look polished and capable and so feel super-confident. A chic style that stays crease- and shine-free throughout the day is essential – leaving you time to get on with more important things.

Unless you are aiming to make a special statement about your individuality, it's advisable to avoid a style of make-up that is too extreme or unusual, but *do* choose positive colours like semi-matte wine red for lips and non-sparkling shades for eyes.

WORK BASICS

Keep your make-up in a clear case, so that you can see things easily and quickly. Look out for mini-lipsticks and buy single eyeshadow palettes so that you can keep your kit as light as possible.

Your kit should include:
● Make-up mirror – look for one that is lightweight, flat and with a cover. Mirrors in compacts always become covered with powder and are often too small.
● Make-up sponge. Hold it in a clear plastic wallet.
● Pressed powder compact with puff.
● Powder brush – ideally a twist-up brush that is held in its own neat case (for removing excess powder).
● Concealer stick.
● Blusher, which can double up as an extra eyeshadow.
● Eye pencil with a sponge tip at one end.
● Smudge-proof brown or black mascara.
● Crease-resistant matte eyeshadow in a soft colour.
● Nail file.
● Hand cream.
● Hairbrush and small pump-action hairspray.

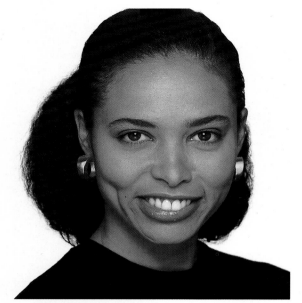

DAY INTO NIGHT

Going out straight from work?
Learn these quick fix-it tips.

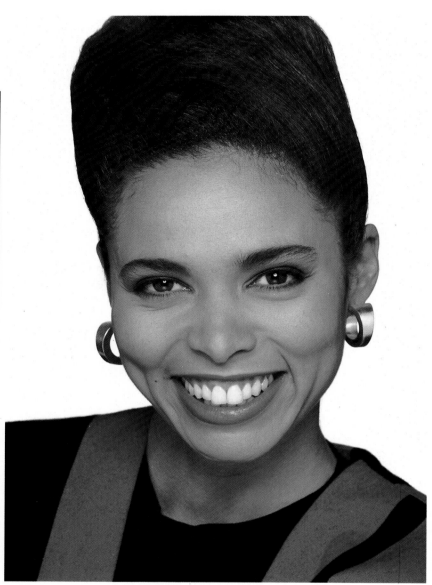

When someone springs the suggestion of an impromptu evening out, or when other commitments mean that you're frantically busy until the moment you're due to head out to a party, use these retouching tips to revive your make-up instantly.

When re-applying make-up, it's a good strategy to use slightly deeper shades than those you used during the day, but aim for a light look. If you apply too much make-up, you may wind up looking tired.

● Blot the T-zone with tissue to remove oils. Gently wipe off your lip colour. Now use a dry make-up sponge to lift off foundation and face powder from your forehead, nose and chin, and blusher from your cheeks. Keep cotton buds with you to smooth eye make-up. Refresh your face by spritzing it with mineral water mist and blot dry.

● Stay with similar but deeper eyeshadow shades compared with those you wore in the day, applying them in a different way to give your face a fresh look. Keep colour above the eye to ensure that you look bright-eyed rather than smoky and sultry which could turn into a heavy-eyed look later in the evening. Emphasize the outer corner of your eyes and apply a paler semi-matte shade as a highlighter just under the brow.

● If your mascara has become clogged, you can solve the problem by holding your lashes gently with your

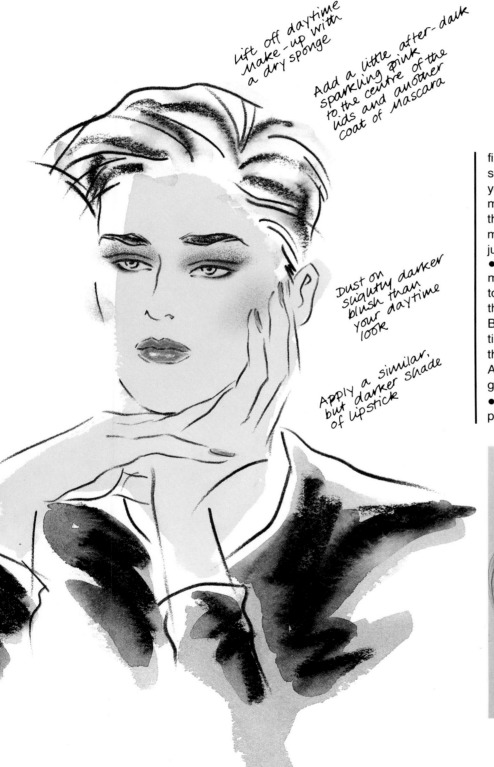

Lift off daytime make-up with a dry sponge

Add a little after-dark sparkling pink to the centre of the lids and another coat of mascara

Dust on slightly darker blush than your daytime look

Apply a similar, but darker shade of lipstick

fingers. Some fibres should come away and you can reapply the mascara to the tips of the lashes only. If the mascara is waterproof, just reapply it.

● Apply a little moisturizer or Vaseline to your lips to soften them ready for lipstick. Blot your lips using a tissue and then outline them with a lip pencil. A bright lip shade will give an instant lift!

● Press on a *little* face powder (use too much and the skin will look clogged).

● Use the same formulation and the same colour-family of blusher as you used in the day. It is unwise to try to apply powder blusher over cream and vice versa.

Remember to check regularly during the evening that your face is not shining, your eyelids are not creased and that your lipstick is not too dry.

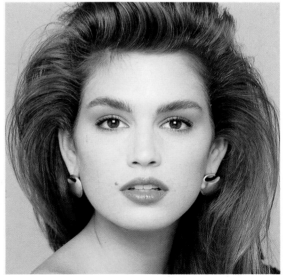

GLAMOROUS NIGHTS

*Discover how to create a stunning evening face –
it's your chance to pull out all the stops!*

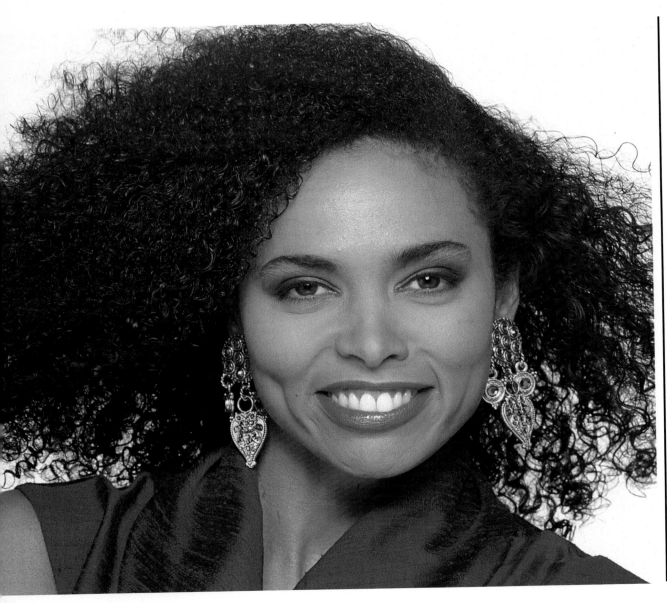

Come the evening, and a special occasion, it's time to make an extra effort. A sexy and vibrant make-up is fun to wear; hot colours such as fuchsia pink and true red look striking on lips while brilliant purple, emerald and royal blue light up eyes.

When you're creating a strong look, begin with a clean, moisturized face and sit in good, even light. When deciding the colours and areas of emphasis, bear in mind the type of light you'll be seen in later – a dark environment will draw the colour from your make-up.

Foundation and powder are essential (unless your skin is tanned), making you look extra glamorous and keeping the colours looking good for longer.

Focus attention on to your eyes. Use coloured liquid

eyeliners or pencils, adding darker colours at the outer corners to lengthen and emphasize your eyes. Coloured mascaras, matched to your eyeliner, are a fast way to a dramatic look.

For stunning evening style, shimmery shadows give extra impact, but avoid them if the skin on your eyelids is very creased since they will only advertise the fact. Gold shadow is a good colour to keep in your make-up box: use it to accent the outer edge of the browbone and sweep it up slightly on to your temples.

Blusher has a major part to play in creating an evening make-up, but never overdo it. You may find it best to complete your make-up, dress and then apply blusher last. If in doubt, use a soft shade rather than a deep one. It is easier to build up colour than to take it down if you decide that you have applied too much.

Using a large brush, dust a little blusher on to your cheeks first, then use the remaining colour on the brush to touch on to the temples, the sides of the forehead and the chin. Take a little more on to the brush and sweep over your cleavage for a subtle boost.

You can position blusher and contour cheeks for precise definition. The compacts that contain two or three shades of blusher are especially useful for evening make-up. If you have a round face, wear blusher higher up on cheekbones and top it with highlighter. Longer faces look dramatic if blusher is placed just below the cheekbones.

Make your lips an exciting feature at night. Try vivid colours such as rich reds or wild, shocking pink.

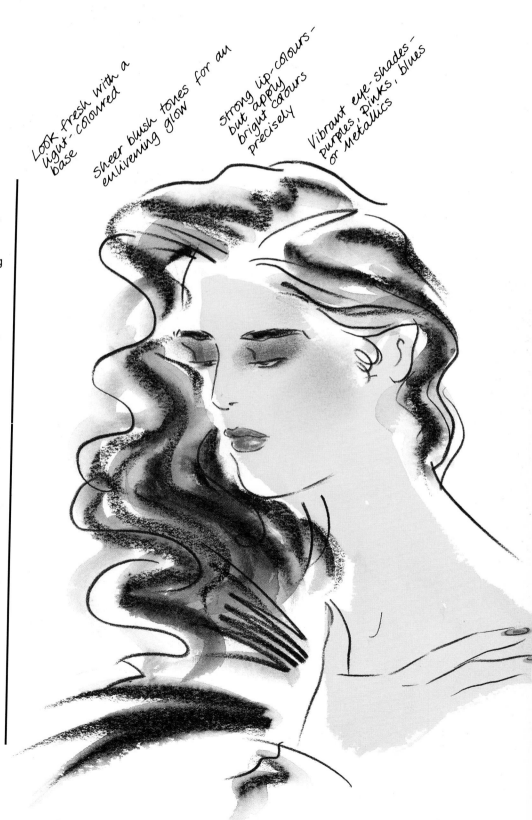

Look fresh with a light-coloured base

Sheer blush tones for an enlivening glow

Strong lip-colours - but apply bright colours precisely

Vibrant eye-shades - purples, pinks, blues or metallics

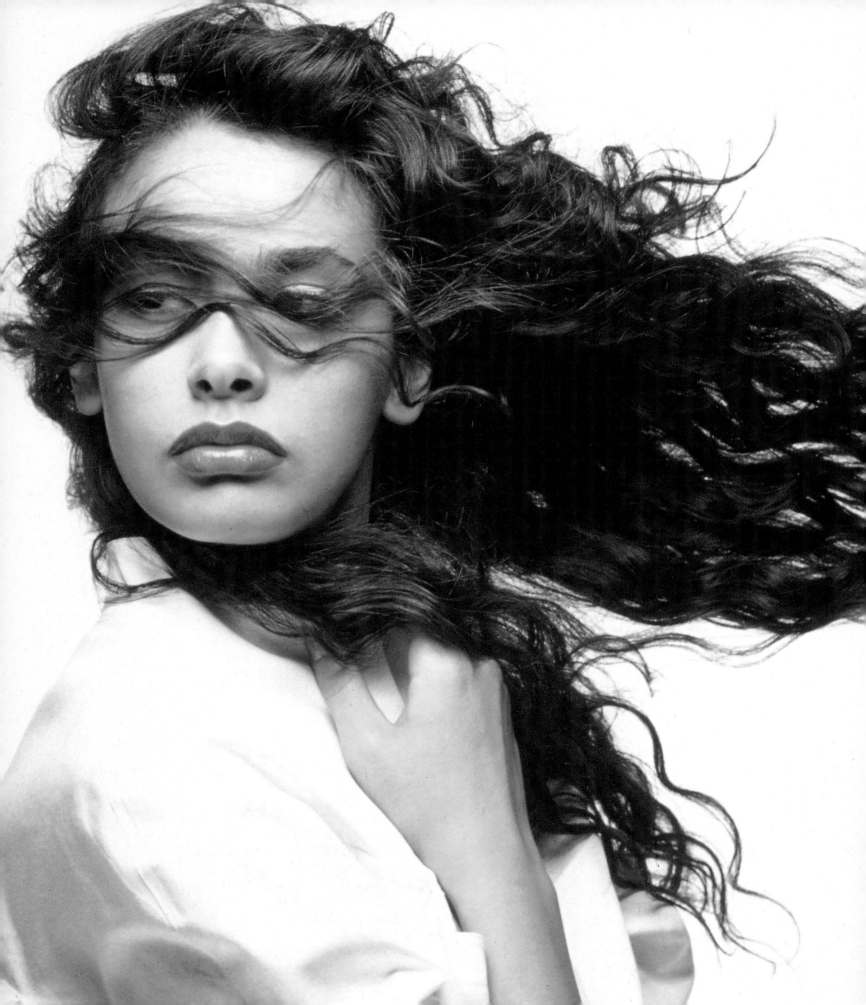

HAIRCARE

Your hair is your most versatile beauty asset.
You can change its style, colour and shape, temporarily or
permanently, often altering your image quite dramatically.
It's important to be aware of your hair type and to look
after your crowning glory accordingly, to keep it
in peak condition. Remember that beautiful hair
is healthy hair, full of bounce and shine.

HAIR BASICS

Wise up on fundamental haircare – it will save you time in the long run.

How you care for your hair will make all the difference to its appearance. Treating it kindly will reward you many times over since it will look naturally beautiful, needing very little extra input of time and effort.

HAIR FACTS

On average hair grows about 2.5 cm (1 in) per month, with the strongest growth period for women being between the ages of 14 and 40, when you also produce the most oestrogen. But your hair never stops growing, it just slows down as you get older.

A strand of hair is made up of three layers, the medulla, cortex and cuticle.

The medulla runs the length of the hair shaft, but is often broken at intervals and sometimes people with fine hair have no medulla at all. Its exact purpose is unknown, though its presence or absence seems to make little difference to what you can do with your hair.

The cortex makes up between seventy-five and ninety per cent of the hair shaft, containing cells that affect the elasticity and strength of your hair and pigments giving it its colour.

The outer layer, the cuticle, is made of flat, overlapping scales that provide a protective covering for the other layers When these scales lie flat, light bounces off them easily, making the hair look shiny.

The hairs grow out of follicles in the scalp, at the base of which lie the papillae. These absorb nutrients from the blood supply. As soon as a new hair surfaces from the follicle, through the skin, the cells die and harden (keratinize). All visible hair is then, in effect, dead.

A DIET FOR YOUR HAIR

A balanced diet benefits your hair as much as the rest of your body, but hair is one of the last in the queue for nutrients, as the vital organs of the body take precedence. Particularly important for healthy hair are the B complex of vitamins, vitamins A and E, proteins, iron and iodine.

SQUEAKY CLEAN AND PROPERLY PROTECTED

It is important to get the basics of haircare – shampooing, conditioning, drying and brushing – right, if you are to avoid problems that will take time to correct later.

Shampoo

Shampoo cleans, but does not repair the hair. Choosing one that works for you is often a trial-and-error process, but there are some useful guidelines:

- Pick a shampoo that is designed for your hair type as this should leave your hair feeling clean and looking shiny (shampoo should not leave any stickiness behind or dull the hair).
- Never use washing-up liquid or household detergent on your hair as they are highly alkaline and disturb your hair's pH balance.
- Avoid having a communal family shampoo – the chances are that everyone will have a different hair type – so buy a selection.
- Change your shampoo every now and then; hair seems to develop a resistance to a shampoo's ingredients after a period of time, sometimes the result of a build-up of styling products.
- Don't throw away a shampoo that doesn't seem to lather. The amount of lather produced is determined by the active level of detergent used in the shampoo and does not influence its cleansing ability – it is more a cosmetic touch.

Rinse well for shiny hair

Always rinse your hair thoroughly in clean, warm water to eliminate any remaining shampoo and conditioner. If traces of these are left in the hair they make it look dull and feel sticky, and also leave particles that flake from the scalp like dandruff.

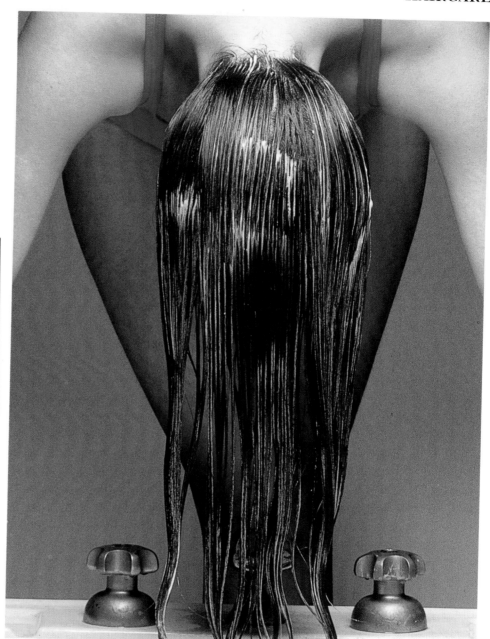

Conditioner

Conditioners cannot *mend* damaged hair but they can help prevent damage getting worse and protect the hair by leaving a film on the cuticle. They have the effect of flattening the cuticle, which makes light reflect off it so your hair looks wonderfully shiny. Conditioner also works to untangle your hair – especially useful if your hair is over–processed and so tends to be knotty.

● Use conditioner after every shampoo (on the whole of your head if your hair is dry or just the ends if it is oily) – it shouldn't leave your hair lank unless you do not rinse it properly.

● Avoid products that claim to shampoo and condition in one because the functions of *washing* and *protecting* are different and cannot really be successfully combined.

● Apply only a small amount of conditioner as your hair won't absorb any surplus and it will take longer to rinse out.

Drying without damage

Let your hair dry naturally as often as possible. With a towel, blot, don't rub the hair. When using a hairdryer point it down the hair shaft to keep the cuticle flat. Do not brush or comb wet hair more than is necessary – it is very vulnerable.

Choosing combs

When buying a comb, check that it has a smooth join down the centre. Uneven jagged plastic will damage the hair shaft. The best option is a comb that is 'sawcut' in one piece with wide, rounded teeth.. Trichologists normally recommend avoiding metal combs which can cause damage.

HAIR TYPING

Knowing your hair type and caring for its particular needs is the first step to a crowning glory.

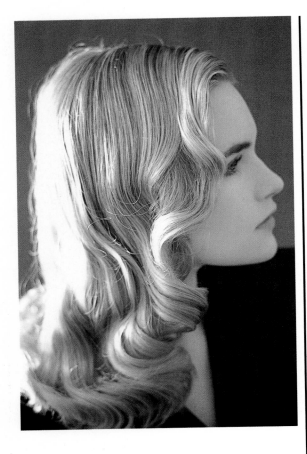

Recognizing your hair type will ensure that you give it the best possible care. There are many factors which will affect your natural hair type and alter the needs of your hair.

DRY AND/OR DAMAGED

The causes of this can be:
- Heredity.
- The use of too many harsh chemical treatments, such as bleaching, or incorrect use or over-use of hair dryers or heated rollers.
- Over-exposure to the sun, sea or chlorinated water.
- Not using conditioner.

Haircare
- Shampoo and condition with moisturizing products two to three times a week, but if you prefer to wash your hair every day, use a mild shampoo and a lighter conditioner.
- Give your hair a deep conditioning treatment once a week.
- Let your hair dry naturally as often as possible, but if you have to use a hair dryer, set it on a low speed and temperature.
- Don't use at-home perming or bleaching kits as your hair could become even more damaged – go to a salon for professional advice.
- Wear a bathing cap if you go swimming and a hat, scarf or special hair-protecting product in the sun.
- Foods high in protein such as fish, poultry and pulses will help combat brittle hair.
- Massage your scalp gently to improve the circulation and stimulate the sebaceous glands which produce the body's own natural conditioner for hair – sebum.

OILY

This can have several causes, including:
- Heredity.
- High hormonal activity.
- Under- or over-washing using harsh products.
- Brushing too frequently which over-stimulates the sebaceous glands in the scalp.

Haircare
- Use a comb rather than a brush and don't style or touch your hair more than is necessary, to avoid stimulating the sebaceous glands.
- Use a mild shampoo, washing your hair as often as necessary, and use a conditioner designed for oily hair, but only on the ends.
- Give your hair a final rinse with a little lemon or vinegar added to the water as this restores the pH balance of your hair.
- Avoid wearing hats

or scarves as they may make the problem worse.
• Check that your diet is healthy and balanced.

COMBINATION HAIR

This combination of greasy scalp with dry ends can be caused by:
• Chemical treatments such as perming and bleaching.
• Not having your hair trimmed frequently enough; approximately every six weeks is usually recommended.

Haircare

• As for oily hair, use a comb in preference to a brush.
• Shampoo your scalp only; when you rinse out the shampoo it will run down the hair shaft, cleaning it in the process.
• Try alternating shampoos for dry and greasy hair.
• Use conditioner only on the ends of your hair, not the scalp.

NORMAL

It is very rare and lucky to have completely normal hair.

Normal hair is the result of sensible haircare, regular trims, few, if any, chemical treatments, and a good diet. Oh, and good genes!

Haircare

• Keep to your usual haircare routine and trims to maintain its good condition.
• Use conditioner to protect the ends and use an occasional deep-conditioning treatment.
• Try to avoid damaging your hair with too much chemical processing.

AFRO HAIR

Afro hair has curved follicles, which give it its characteristic springy curl. The hair strands are deceptively thin and are actually fewer in number per square

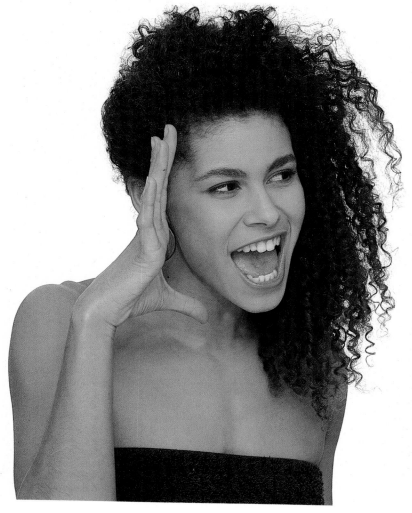

centimetre than other hair types. As a result, Afro hair is particularly vulnerable to damage during chemical processes.

Many people with this hair type have their hair straightened, but it is a technically very complicated process and can cause terrible damage to the hair's infrastructure, leading to hair loss unless treated professionally. Do not use at-home straightening kits.

This hair type is invariably dry, as its very structure makes it difficult for sebum from the sebaceous glands to travel down the hair shaft.

Haircare

• Massaging a little specially blended hair oil into the hair after shampooing and conditioning helps to alleviate dryness.
• If you have a mixed hair type, with a greasy scalp and dry ends, avoid using too many oils as they may block the hair follicles. Instead, shampoo minimally and use conditioner only on the ends of your hair, not on the scalp.
• Braiding looks great on ethnic hair, but you should not keep your hair in this style for long periods, as the constant pulling on the scalp exerts too much pressure on the hair follicles and can lead to hair loss.

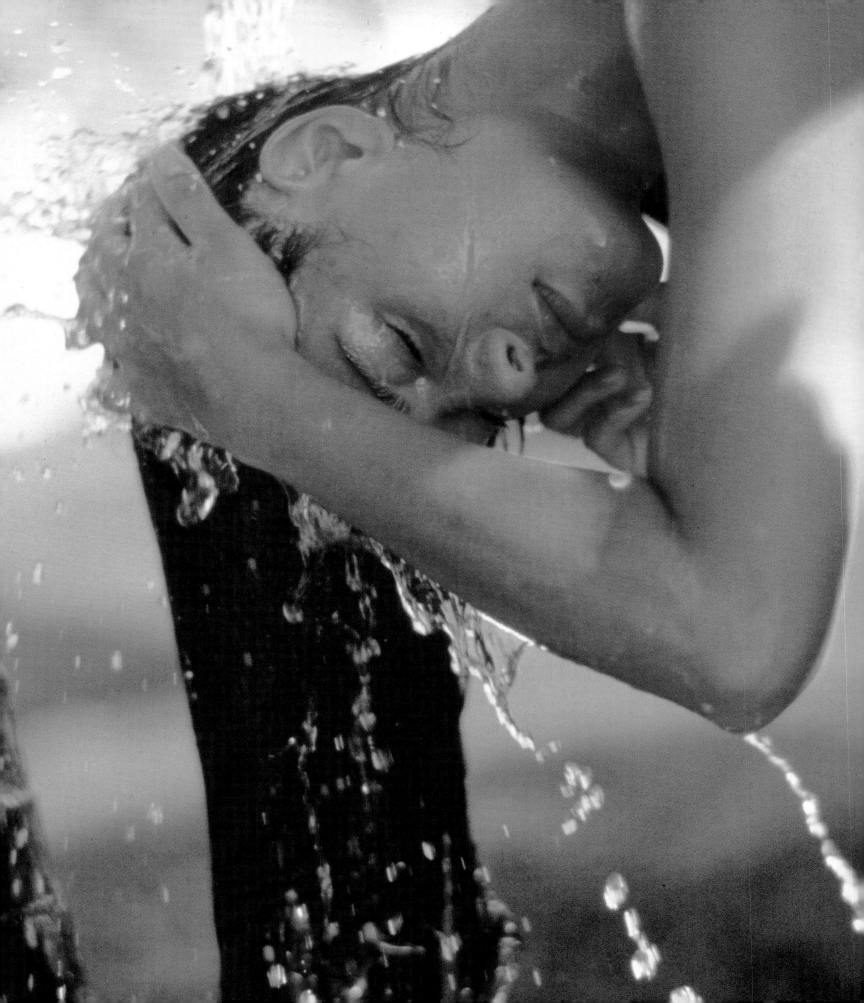

HAIR PROBLEMS

If your hair is looking less than its best,
it's time for some special treatment.

Three of the most common complaints about hair are dullness, thinning and dandruff. These conditions may have any of several causes and there are a number of different treatments to try.

DULL HAIR
This may be caused by:
- stress
- not rinsing out shampoo and conditioner properly
- a build-up of the residue of styling products
- sun damage
- chemical treatments
- heated drying or styling appliances.

Treatment
- Rinse with white wine vinegar after shampooing and before conditioning.
- Dry your hair correctly (page 99).
- Protect your hair in the sun with lotions containing sunscreens, or wear a hat.
- Avoid chemical treatments until your hair has recovered.

THINNING HAIR
Hair loss can be caused by:
- stress
- hormonal changes
- poor diet
- heredity
- pulling the hair while brushing or scraping it back too often into tight pony tails.

Treatment
- Massage your scalp daily to stimulate hair growth.
- Condition your hair – it coats and thus thickens the hair shaft and has the cosmetic effect of making your hair look fuller.
- Hormone therapy has been proven to help hereditary hair loss so check with your doctor if you've tried everything else.

Adding volume
A time-saving trick for increasing volume on chin-to-shoulder-length hair can be done before you put on your make-up or have your breakfast.

When your hair is damp, section it all over and twist each section into small buns. Secure the sections with covered elastic bands (rubber bands damage your hair) or hair pins, so that you end up with about ten 'knots' covering the head. When your hair is dry, remove the elastics or pins and brush or shake through.

DANDRUFF
Dandruff is a non-inflammatory scaling of the scalp. Most hair specialists (trichologists) refer to it simply as scaling. Possible causes include:
- An increase in normal cell turnover, which is very often the result of stress or a reaction to dairy products.
- Flaking due to a

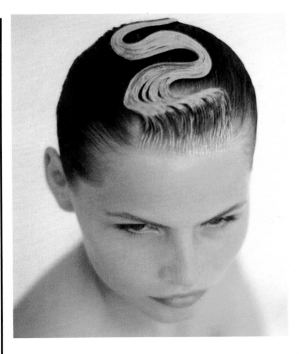

disturbance in the intercellular 'cement' of the cortex and cuticle of the hair – usually a result of lack of moisture. This is a less common cause. Sometimes harsh shampoos can cause this intercellular cement to dissolve.

Treatment
- Shampoo frequently with a mild shampoo (shampoos containing zinc pyrithione help, but tend to dry the hair shaft and should not be used on an inflamed scalp).
- Cut dairy products out of your diet for a while to see if this is a cause in your case.
- Visit a trichologist if the problem persists or if you experience redness and irritation.

CUTTING CLEVER

A good cut is the basis of a great hair-style and will keep your hair in top condition.

The hair-style you choose can make all the difference to whether you feel confident and happy with your appearance or uneasy and dissatisfied. It is important, therefore, to find a hairdresser with whom you can develop a good rapport and who can reflect your personality in your hair-style.

A stylist will adapt a cut according to your hair type and the directions of hair growth, and ensure that the style will enhance your features and flatter the shape of your face. A stylist will also take your life-style into account and should ask you questions like: 'How busy are you? Do you have time to spend styling your hair in the morning or do you rush out with it still damp? Do you like using styling products such as mousse or gel?'.

It's a good idea to show your hairdresser photographs of styles that appeal to you, so that you can be advised as to whether they will work with your hair. Some salons nowadays have high-tech computers which take a photograph of you and then project hundreds of different styles and hair colours on to the image at the touch of a button. The hairdresser will select styles from the computer's memory banks that are workable for your hair type. These computers are a fast and useful styling tool which could inspire you to try a style you never dreamed would suit you.

A clever haircut is one that will look good simply blow-dried, and one that is versatile enough to allow you to change the style with ease.

Regular cuts

You should have your hair cut approximately every six weeks, although a very precise, short style may require shaping as often as every four weeks.

Changing hairdresser

If you are considering trying a new hairdresser, book in for a simple service such as a trim before plunging in for a major change of style. This way you can find out if the hair-stylist thinks the same way you do and it will give them the chance to get to know your hair and your individual requirements.

Do be open to new ideas from your stylist. Changing your hair-style is the most effective way to inject new energy into your look.

SHORT CUTS

A top salon that specializes in short haircuts advises its clients: 'Short styles save you time and keep you looking terrific whatever the environmental conditions – in humid heat and high winds'.

Short hair can be cut and styled to create many different looks: sharp, angular styles look strong and individual, while there are soft wavy styles that are modern classics. The added bonus with short hair is that it can look professional and smart in an instant.

Hot brushes and tongs are a fast way to give short hair a lift. Keep a cordless styler in your bag or desk drawer so that you can change your style before you go out for the evening.

Versatile bobs

The classic short bob remains modern-looking and is easy to style and wear. Blunt cut on straight hair the bob looks chic and shiny. You can use flattening irons to keep hair that tends to wave slightly straight and sleek. A short bob to just below the ears looks young and fun.

Layering a bob gives the effect of movement. A layered bob can be worn full and wide, scrunch-dried and teased out with the aid of mousse, or close to the face, with the sides swept forwards. A permed bob with a straight fringe is a new variation on the theme.

Your hairdresser will advise you as to whether a side parting or a fringe is best for you. Asymmetric cuts work well on the bob shape and add an element of individuality.

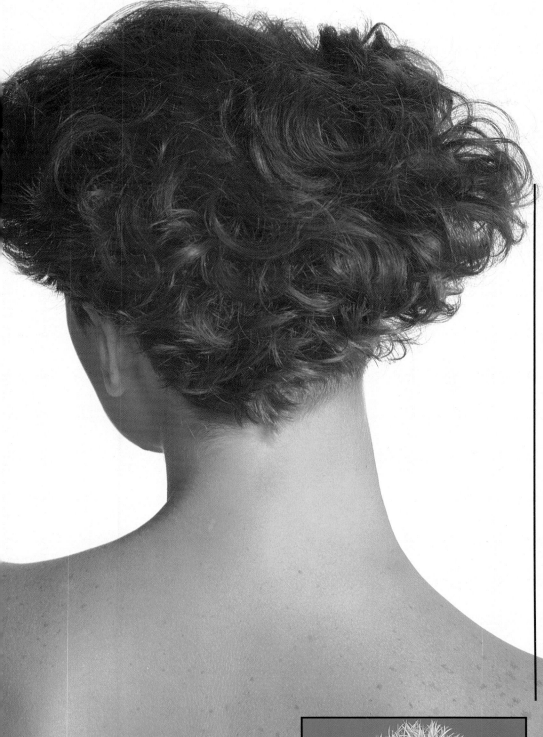

The urchin look

Gamine cuts that are short, layered and cut close to the head look especially chic when they are worn slightly tousled. Boyish-looking, the contrast between the short, short hair and a pretty face beneath is appealing and will attract attention!

Short and sharp

Razor cuts and sharp, spiked styles are androgynous in concept, the styles often mirroring those worn by male contemporaries. These cuts are often graduated through the sides of the hair and at the nape of the neck. Although they require minimal styling, they do demand regular cutting to keep them looking good. Many women head for the local barber to get their crop. It's a good idea to leave some length on top, as this will increase the versatility of your style, particularly if you have thick hair with a good texture.

Classic waves

If a waved style is more you, consider having a soft perm or invest in a wave maker. These resemble crimpers, and will make gentle, rippling 'marcel waves' through your hair.

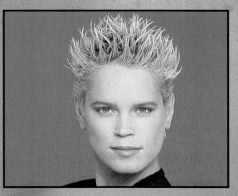

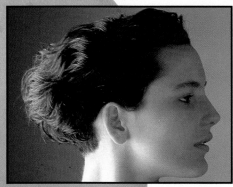

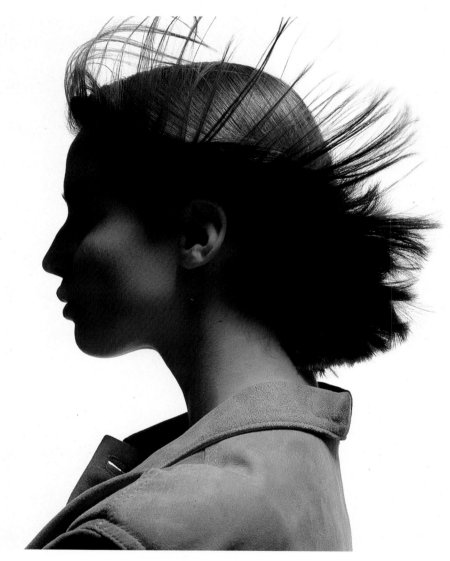

MID-LENGTH AND LONG HAIR

Whether one-length and sleek, or layered and full, longer hair can make you feel especially glamorous. The length of your hair should be determined by your face and by your height: for instance, long hair can look unbalanced on women who are not very tall. The length is also governed by the growth rate of your hair (some hair will never grow very long) and by your hair type – if your hair looks lank and lies too flat against your head, it may be that the weight of the hair is pulling it down, so try a shorter cut.

It is essential to keep longer hair in top condition – always keep brushing to the minimum and do it gently. Have it cut regularly so that split ends don't have a chance to develop – they work their way up the length of the hair if left to do so. Find a hairdresser who is prepared to spend time trimming off split ends along the length of the hair – twisting the hair in small sections at a time and then snipping off any stray ends.

Fringe appeal

Consider keeping interest at the front if your hair is long. A fringe can be short and straight (which looks sassy and strong) or longer for a pretty finish. A layered fringe will enable you to create fullness. Layer your hair through the sides and you will frame the face with soft, feathery wisps of hair.

Volume with length

If you want to wear your hair long, but like height on top, there are two options open to you: a 'no curl' permanent wave just at the roots will give hair volume and make it easier to style. Recently developed, short-term body builders give gentle wave and body which last six weeks. Stylers are twisted into the roots and the lotion applied. Half an hour later the stylers are removed.

The other possibility for giving volume and interest to long hair is heated stylers. Hot brushes can be used to curl under or flick out the ends on a shoulder-length blunt cut. Alternatively, heated styling sticks can be twisted into the top of the hair to give a fast fillip.

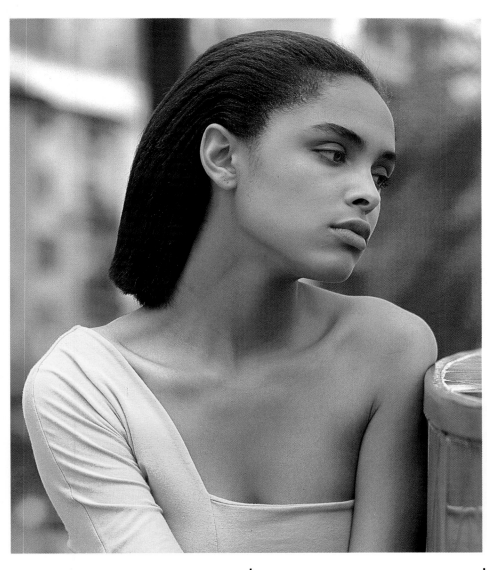

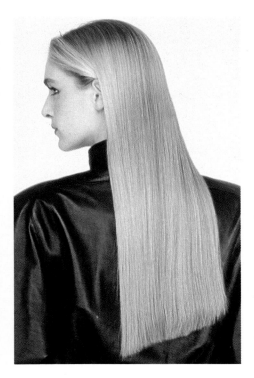

Romantic curls

Ringlets make a romantic look that can be created with tongs or by sleeping with your hair in rags. Twist a lock of your hair and wind it round your finger. Insert the end of a strip of fabric through the hole created by your finger and fasten it with a knot. Long-lasting ringlets can be achieved with a spiral perm. As a variation, the top layer of hair can be wound into ringlets which then rest on top of straight hair.

Hair extensions

If you are frustrated by trying to grow your hair long, or are trying to grow out layers, extensions are a clever method of adding instant length. The 'monofibre' extensions used can be realistically coloured or chosen to contrast with your own hair shade for a frankly fake, fun look. Extensions are heat-sealed on to the hair – this does not damage your hair and the plastic seal can be twisted off later.

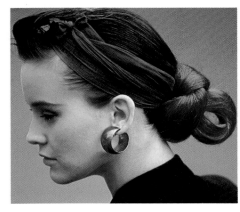

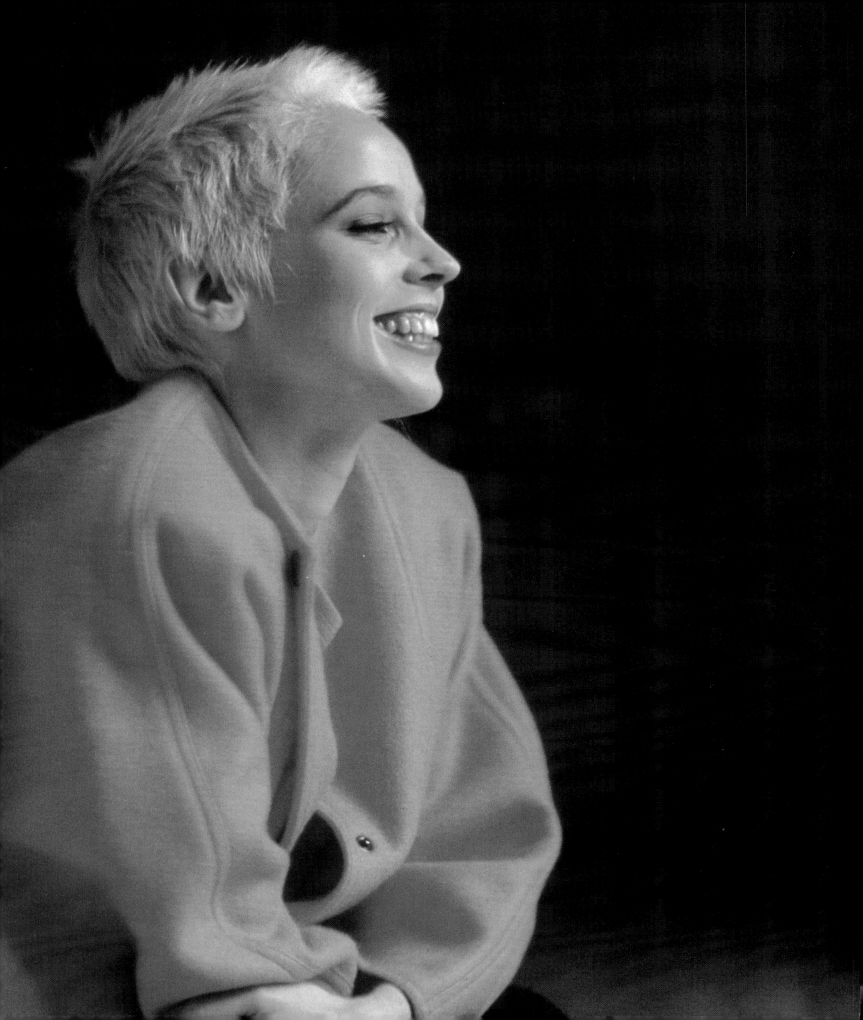

COLOUR SENSE

Colouring is one of the quickest ways to change your image.
Check out all the options to find the best method for your hair.

Before you make any changes to the colour of your hair, think about your colouring, features, age and even your occupation. Remember too, that what looks great on someone else may not suit you.

It's a good idea to try on a few wigs in colours and styles that you are thinking of – particularly if you are contemplating a dramatic change. Alternatively, some salons have a specialized computer that can show you images of yourself with different tones in your hair.

If you want a more permanent colour change, rather than just a rinse, do go to a salon. An expert colourist will examine your hair and make *realistic* suggestions, taking your hair's health, porosity and natural colour into consideration, as hair colours react differently on various types and conditions of hair.

There are several different colouring techniques. Listed below are the most commonly used, what they do and how long they last. However, colouring technology is advancing so much year by year, it's worth asking your local salon what they have to offer.

Colourways

For the most natural-looking effects, just choose a shade or two lighter or darker than your natural colour. Extremes of colour work best on people who are very confident and well co-ordinated.

TINTING

This is usually a blend of a tint and hydrogen peroxide which penetrates the cortex and then is sealed in. The tint combines with your natural hair colour to produce the final shade.

● Going a few shades *lighter* seems to work better than going *darker*, which can look flat and matte.
● In a salon, tell them the history of your hair as it may affect how the ' tint takes; the initial treatment is always more expensive than later retouching treatments, so it is important to get it right.
● At home, don't attempt to use a tint on previously bleached hair in the hope of improving the colour – it will probably end up brassy.
● After tinting, be sure to condition your hair regularly.
● Tinting will normally need retouching every month or so, depending on how different it is from your natural colour.

BLEACHING

Bleach tends to be ammonia-based (though there are ammonia-free varieties), mixed with hydrogen peroxide. It removes the natural pigment; a blonde toner then gives it the characteristic colour.

● Bleaching damages the hair so badly that it's best to resort to it only if you can't achieve blonde with a few shades of tint.
● It is expensive and time-consuming to return to your natural colour if you find that you don't like your hair bleached blonde.
● Salon bleaching always looks better than home-bleached hair.
● Your hair will need retouching, which not only means frequent visits to the salon, but each re-application of bleach damages your hair further.

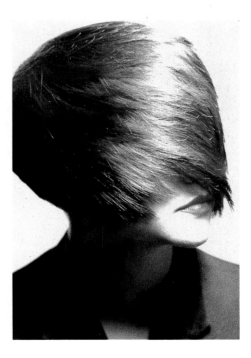

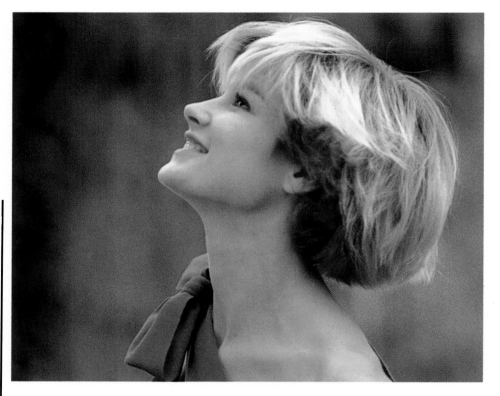

TEMPORARY COLOUR RINSES

These colour the hair by coating the cuticle and wash out quickly. They normally shampoo-in, but you can buy them in the form of setting lotions.
● Your hair colour is not dramatically changed; rinses just add depth.
● The condition of your hair is not affected, unless the rinse contains a built-in conditioner.
● Rinses can be used on all non-processed hair, though they work best on fair hair.
● They are cheap, quick and easy to use at home.

SEMI-PERMANENT COLOUR

These, logically, are not as permanent as a tint, but more lasting than a rinse, penetrating the cuticle only.
● Like rinses, semi-permanent colours don't produce a dramatic change unless you choose a dark shade and your natural colour is blonde, and so can be used just to brighten your own hair colour.
● There's little regrowth problem with this method as the colour fades out after about six to eight washes.
● Semi-permanent colour is reasonably cheap and easy in the salon or at home.

HIGHLIGHTING OR STREAKS

These are done by using a peroxide or tint mix that penetrates the hair cortex, applied by either the foil or cap method. Foil is usually more expensive but gives better results; pulling strands through a perforated rubber cap is cheaper and, if done well, can look very natural.
● Highlighting is kinder than total bleaching; although it still damages your hair (sometimes leading to it knotting easily and becoming frizzy), it *can* look wonderful, like naturally sun-streaked hair, giving the impression of depth and movement.
● It is a technique best left to the salon, as there is too much room for mistakes with home kits.
● On average, highlights will need to be redone every three months or so, though more frequent retouching may be necessary.

VEGETABLE COLOURS

These are colourants that use natural ingredients such as camomile or henna.
● They add colour, depth and shine.
● They are fairly cheap and completely harmless.
● They can be used both at home and in the salon, although they tend not to work on grey hair unless they are specially designed for it, and highlighted and bleached hair may go a little orange.
● The colour fades out gradually.

Colour care
● *Don't expose coloured hair to the sun as it will probably change its shade. Wear a hat or specialized hair protector.*
● *Colouring often makes your hair look thicker, saving time on styling. Be sure to condition it regularly.*

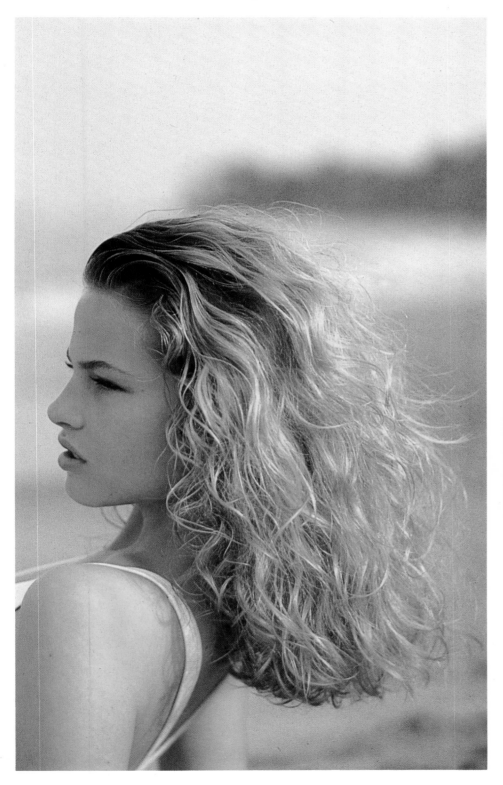

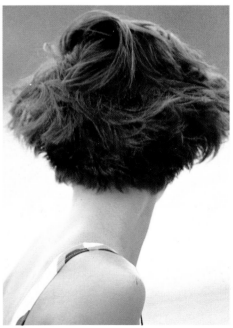

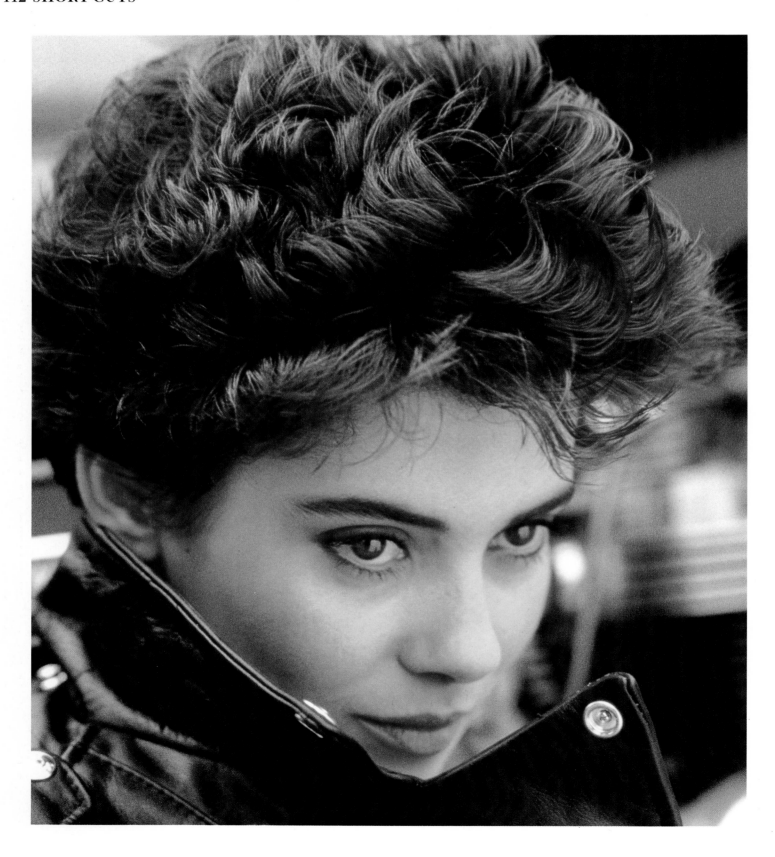

PERMANENT SOLUTIONS

Whether you want cascading curls or just a little extra volume,
a perm will inject vitality into your hair-style.

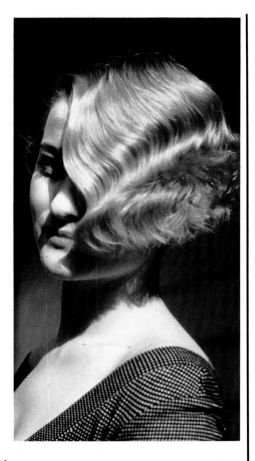

Perms are terrific time-savers as far as styling is concerned, and nowadays they are so versatile that they can be used in a variety of ways to give quite different effects. A root perm, for example, will just give lift and body to the hair without waving or curling it.

As perming is a complicated technical process, it is wisest to have it done professionally. Apart from the mishaps you can have with home kits (uneven waves, at worst a dried-out mess) you have no come-back if you have done it yourself.

PRE-PERM POINTERS

● Most people with previously unprocessed hair can have their hair permed successfully. There are perms specifically designed for bleached and highlighted hair, on which your hairdresser can advise you. If your hair is semi-permanently coloured, a suitable perm is usually straightforward. Other kinds of coloured hair should ideally be left for a couple of weeks before perming, to avoid altering the colour. It is usually best to have colouring done *after* a perm.

● Don't have your hair permed if it's not in tip-top condition. Your hairdresser will probably suggest a course of cutting and conditioning treatments with the perming following after a few months.

● If your hair is either very fine or porous, ask in your salon about acid-balanced perms as these have a gentler formulation.

● Consider how different you will look. If you are not happy with a colour, this can be corrected (with time and money); with the perm you asked for, there's little a hairdresser can do. The curl will loosen up in a few weeks, but if you really hate it, your only option may be to have it all cut out.

THE PERMING PROCESS

This involves winding the hair on to rollers (their size and usage depending on the size and type of curl or wave you want) and applying a chemical to break down the hair fibre in the cortex to prepare it for the shape the curler will create. Following the reaction, the hair is rinsed and a neutralizer applied to re-form the hair to hold its curl.

POST-PERM TIPS

● Avoid brushing permed hair as this will create static and separate the curls. Use a wide-toothed comb instead.

● Try to leave a perm for forty-eight hours before shampooing, as the chemicals may still be active.

● If your perm seems to drop slightly, spritz it with a water spray to revive the bounce.

● Condition the roots and ends of your hair regularly to keep it soft.

● Your hairdresser will advise you on how long your perm is likely to last. Depending on the length of your hair, it will probably be three to six months.

SHAPE AND STYLE

Get to grips with gels, mousses, lotions and pomades and you'll discover exciting new styling possibilities for your hair.

The new generation of styling aids has revolutionized haircare and styling. Now we can inject life into our hair by building body and boosting shine in just a few minutes. The new stylers make it possible to control and shape our hair, changing the style from sleek and straight to wild and full in no time at all.

Mousse

This is a fabulous, instant volume builder. It coats the hair making it easier to control and is especially useful for taming frizzy hair and for shaping the curl in permed hair. It will give energy to fine hair and extra texture to straight hair. Many mousses contain conditioners, which are excellent for dry ends.

Apply mousse by squeezing a golfball-sized knob of foam into the palm of your hand and then applying it with your fingers to the roots. Mousse is best applied to slightly damp hair because it will distribute better. Don't be tempted to use too much or you will overload the hair, and be careful to use very little on fine hair or you could end up with a sticky, heavy result.

Experiment with different strengths of mousse. It is often best to buy a mousse with a high hold factor and use less of it than to apply more of a lighter mousse.

If your hair feels lank later in the day, spraying with a little water will revive it. Shape your hair with your fingers as it dries.

Gels

Gel defines texture on curly hair and will sleek and hold straight hair in place. There are several ways to use it. Gel can be applied to wet hair, combed into shape and then left to set hard. Or you can blow-dry the gelled hair, which gives lots of body and bounce but still leaves it looking silky and natural. Gel spreads more easily when applied to wet or slightly damp hair.

Gels formulated for use on dry hair are good for controlling small areas of hair and for slicking it back at the sides of your face. If the brand you are using becomes flaky when you touch or comb your hair, switch to another formulation.

You can combine products such as mousses and gels or mousses and hairspray for extra styling strength.

Styling lotions for blow-drying

These spray-in lotions protect hair from the drying effects of heat when it is blow-dried. They also help to keep the hair cuticle flat, which prevents flyaway ends and increases shine. Many blow-styling formulations will also help to increase the volume of your hair.

Sculpting lotions

These ultra-strong hair shapers are designed to be applied either to damp hair, which is then blow-dried into shape, or to dry hair for fullness or uplifting effects. Use them at the front and sides to create width and on short, spiky hair to make your hair stand straight up!

Hairspray

You can use hairspray for localized styling and to keep your hair sleek. Hairspray holds a polished finish, but allows movement (which sculpting lotions do not). If you simply want to control a few stray ends, spray a little hairspray on to your brush and sweep it through your hair.

Hairspray is indispensable when the atmosphere is humid because it prevents the dampness from making your hair limp. Keep a mini hairspray in your bag – many pump sprays are refillable.

Pomade and wax

These are useful for thick hair, but should not be used on fine hair. Apply a little, using your fingertips to separate and define the hair – for instance, on a spiky fringe. Pomade and wax are terrific for creating shine and for controlling afro hair. Remember that they need to be washed out very thoroughly.

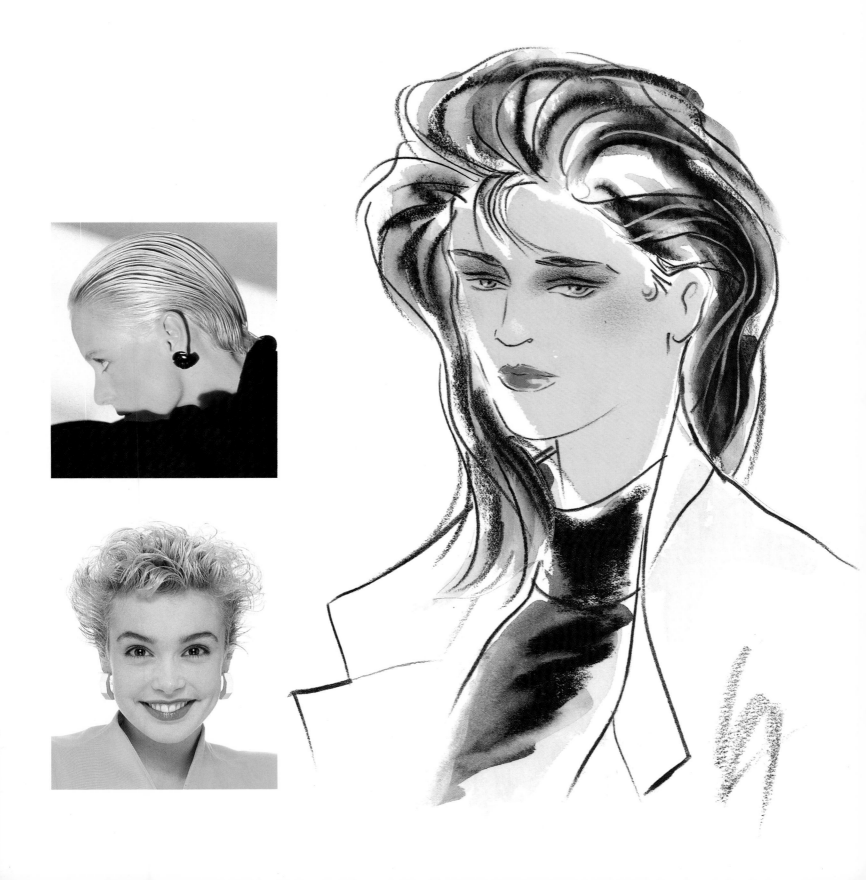

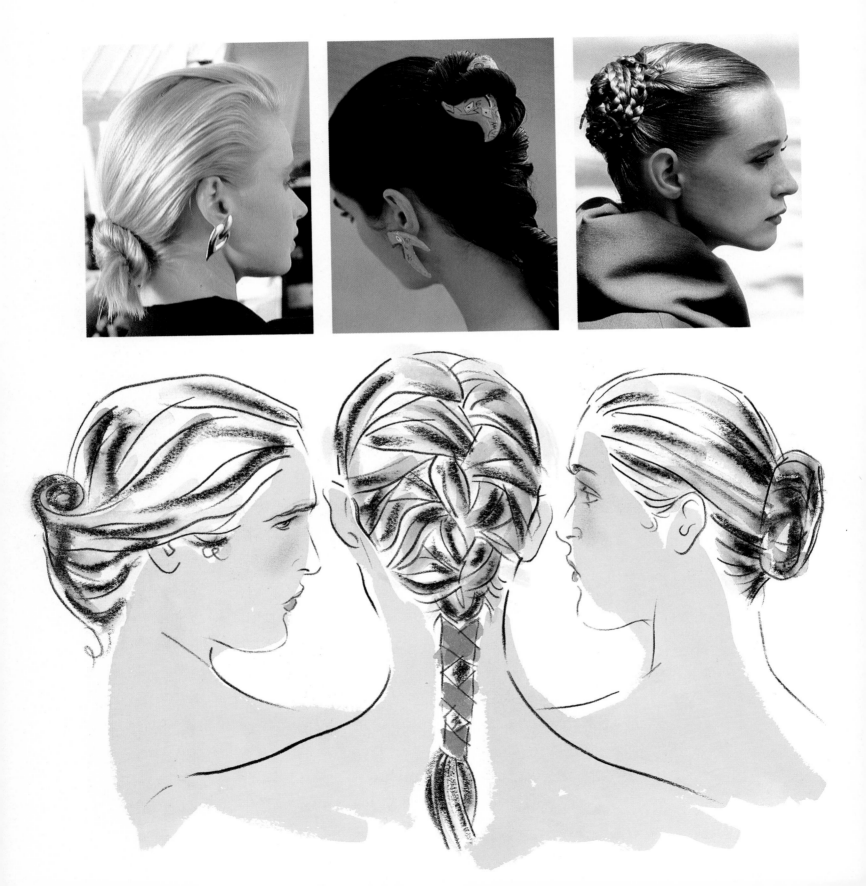

TWISTS, PLAITS AND ROLLS

Modern classicism is today's way with hair looks. There are a multitude of stylish ways to dress mid-length and long hair.

In the same way that we choose accessories to accent a particular outfit, we should consider our hair in terms of what we are going to wear. A hair-style should always tie in with the overall look.

The beauty of mid-length and long hair is that it can be styled in an exciting variety of ways. Twists, plaits, braids, rolls and chignons all look super-stylish and can be worn with simple accessories to secure them in place, or decorated ornately to create knock-out looks.

The key to success when styling is to apply a little mousse or gel to control flyaway ends and to sleek your hair before you start. You need to have a selection of long hairpins, Kirby grips and covered elastics.

Twists

Quick to do, twists can be left soft and natural-looking – there is no need to plaster them with hairspray!

Simply twist your hair along the side of your head on one side and fasten it at the back with a hair-clip.

Now twist back the other side and clip the two pieces together so that the hair hangs sleek and straight behind, or interweave the two twists at the nape of the neck and fasten with long hairpins.

Twists look pretty when several tortoiseshell chignon pins are placed around the twist.

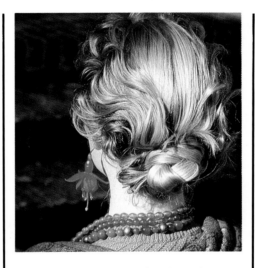

Combs can be used to help hold twists in place. Look for combs without rough edges. Place them in your hair so that they grip by pushing the teeth up towards the crown of the head, then turn the comb and push it down.

Plaits and braids

Ideally you need to have hair of one length to plait and braid it quickly. Practice makes perfect plaits.

Braids (French plaits) are more tricky to do. Starting just below the crown of your head, divide the centre of your hair into three sections, plait these together and then pick up another section on either side of the centre piece and plait together again. Continue down to the nape of your neck and then plait as usual, fastening with a slide or covered elastic at the end.

Rolls and French pleats

Sharp, stylish and with a touch of formality, rolls are fun to wear with clothes that echo the style of the 1940s and 50s.

For a French pleat, take your hair back into the nape of the neck, twisting along the length of the hair. Roll the twist of hair upwards, turning the ends in, and fasten the pleat in place with plenty of pins.

Chignons

These are good on fine to medium-textured hair but take a little more time on heavier hair.

A low chignon placed at the nape of the neck looks modern. You can twist the hair and knot it, pulling the ends through the knot and securing with pins. Alternatively, you can take the hair into a low pony-tail, secure it with a covered elastic and then twist and pin into place.

Look out for hanky knots. These are specially shaped pieces of fabric (raw silk ones look particularly good) which have an elasticated piece at one end. Simply place the fabric over the chignon and twist the elastic around twice to secure it.

HAIR ACCESSORIES

*Read our glossary of terrific hair accessories –
the fastest way to add polish to your look.*

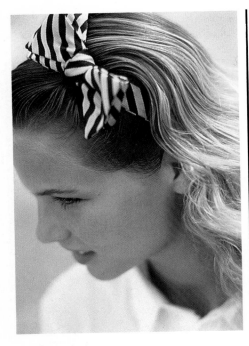

Every season sees a greater variety of hair accessories in the shops. The wide array of beautiful designs is irresistible! A covetable hair accessory will pull together even the simplest outfit.

Hairbands

These are the quickest way to hold mid-length and long hair in place. They are good, too, for days when your hair feels lank because a hairband will keep your hair away from your face and prevent you from touching it. Hairbands made of grosgrain are a good investment since they look smart in the day and chic for the evening.

Slides, clips and barettes

These range from slim gold clips to wide, patterned barettes and shaped metal slides. Look out for classic designs in materials such as bronze titanium, matte black plastic and beaten silver.

Hair-stylists sometimes place gold slides in rows through the hair, positioned 1–2 cm (½–1 in) apart, which looks very effective.

Fabric puffs on elastic

Coloured fabric puffs are the shortest cut to high-impact style. Use brightly coloured satin puffs at night and matte silk in navy, red or black for day, twisting them on to your hair at the nape of your neck, or slightly lower down to form a loose pony-tail.

Towelling elastics

These are fun for weekends and for days at the beach. Gather your hair into a half pony-tail and secure with one fluorescent colour, such as lime. Now fasten a hot pink band at the neck and another colour further down if your hair is long. Alternatively, simply twist two bands in different colours on to a single pony-tail.

Bows

Pretty and feminine, bows can be used to fasten a half pony-tail, to decorate the front of a roll and at the nape of the neck. You can personalize bows with beads, pearls, and buttons such as coin buttons, fastened with strong glue or thread.

Banana clips

These are fun for weekends, and useful too since they keep the hair away from the face.

Snoods

Forties-style net snoods hold your hair neatly back. Roll your hair under before slipping it on. Snoods can also be combined with hairbands.

Fabric pieces

Keep lengths of fabric to twist into your hair as a band or to fasten a pony-tail. You can sweep long hair to one side and then fasten it low down with a piece of cloth. Fabrics with ethnic patterns work particularly well.

If you have very long hair, you can wind the fabric around and along the length of the pony-tail, fastening it with covered elastics at either end and then wrapping the loose ends of the fabric around the elastics to hide them from view.

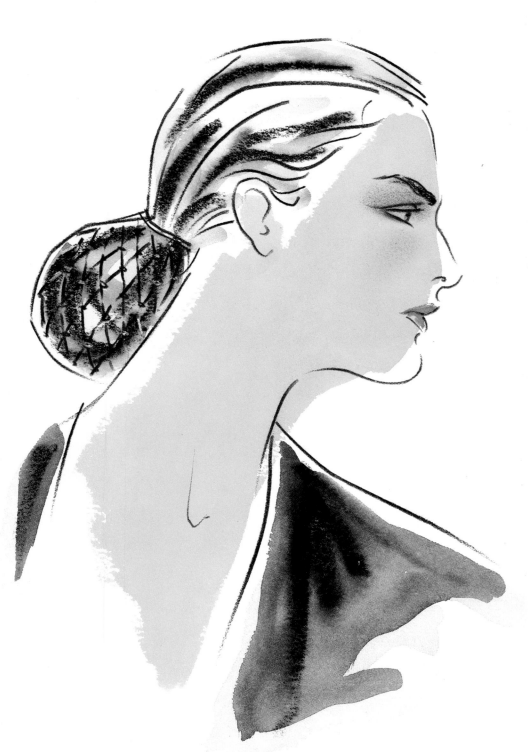

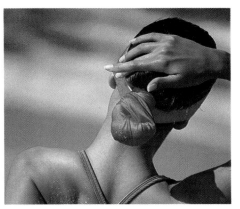

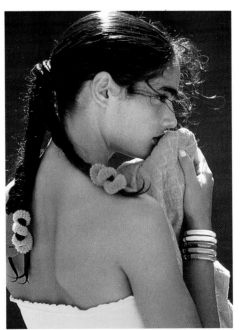

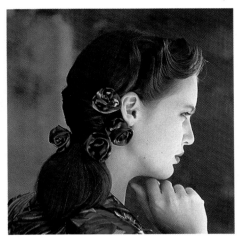

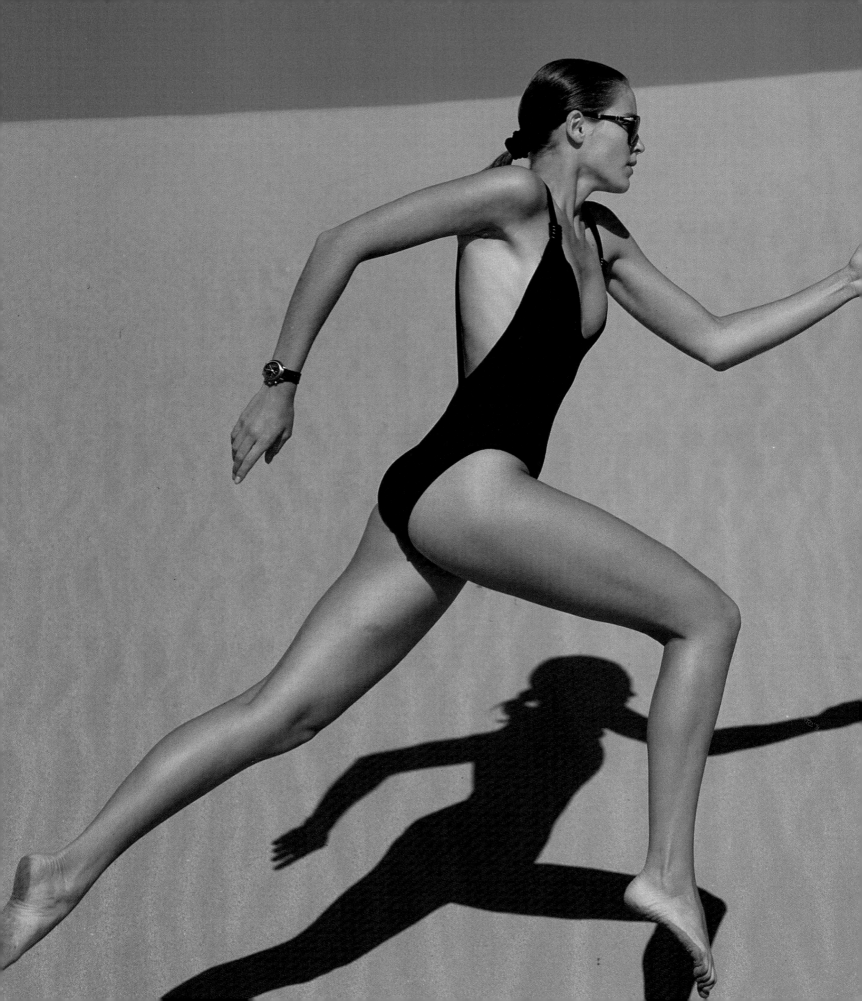

THE BODY BEAUTIFUL

A well-toned body with sleek skin can be achieved through simple exercises and a little regular skincare. By targeting exercise to specific areas you can redefine curves and strengthen muscles — you only need a few spare minutes in your day.

ARM AND SHOULDER SHAPERS

Strong, curvy shoulders and arms will work wonders in balancing your body shape.

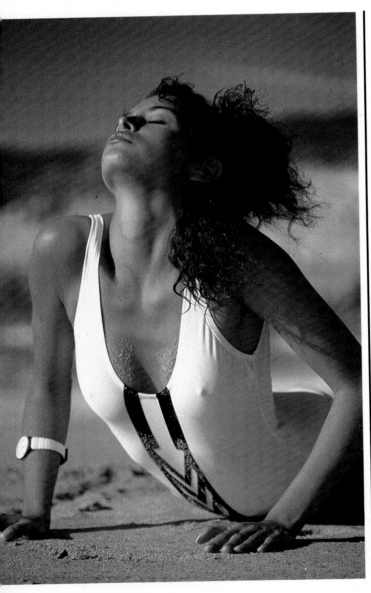

Developing your shoulders makes your waist and hips look at least one size smaller!

You can achieve this by wearing clothes with shoulder pads and by special exercises. Several popular forms of exercise, such as walking, jogging and cycling, either do not tone the upper body at all or tone it only slightly. (Walking with hand-held weights is popular, but be careful if you suspect you may have any underlying cardio-vascular problems, as you are putting extra strain on your heart.)

The arms, especially the backs of arms, benefit greatly from toning exercises geared to this area. Do them every other day and you'll soon be able to carry your suitcase through the airport without the customary struggle.

Swimming is a fast shoulder shaper. However, you should try to include more than one stroke if you are swimming regularly or you could develop problems later on, as muscles may become overdeveloped or inflamed through overuse.

If you play a lot of tennis, be careful – serving incorrectly can lead to swelling and pain. If this happens to you, ask a tennis professional to check your movements and show you how to correct them. Otherwise racquet sports are very good for developing and defining your shoulder contours.

Skincare

Care for the skin on your arms by gently exfoliating (removing dead cells from the surface of the skin, see page 52) with a body scrub or hemp mitt, concentrating on the skin on your elbows and any rough skin on the backs of your upper arms.

Short cuts to pretty elbows

Sit with each elbow in half a lemon for a few minutes to whiten the skin. Then rinse and apply moisturizer.

Weights and exercise

Some exercises involve using weights to increase the amount of work done by your muscles. Use dumbbells (between 1–2kg/ 2–5lb, depending on what weight feels comfortable) or wrist weights.

Warm up

Always warm up your shoulders before starting any sport that uses your arms, using gym equipment and before doing the exercises here.

Raise and lower your shoulders 4 times. Relax your shoulders down.

Push your shoulders back and forwards 4 times.

Circle your arms back 8 times.

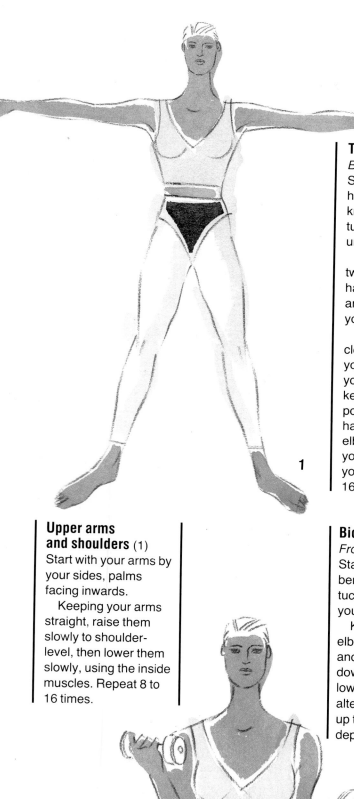

Triceps (3)
Backs of arms
Stand with your feet hip-width apart, your knees slightly bent and tuck your buttocks under well.

Hold either one or two weights with both hands and raise your arms straight above your head.

Keep your arms close to the sides of your head and lower your hands slowly, keeping your elbows pointing up. Raise your hands so that your elbows straighten and your upper arms touch your head. Repeat 8 to 16 times.

Arm and shoulder stretch (5)
Kneel up and place your right arm behind your head with your palm against your back.

With your left hand, gently ease your right elbow inwards so that your hand slides down.

Hold the stretch for 20 seconds, and then repeat with your left arm.

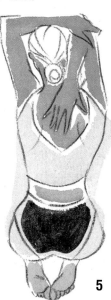

5

Upper arms and shoulders (1)
Start with your arms by your sides, palms facing inwards.

Keeping your arms straight, raise them slowly to shoulder-level, then lower them slowly, using the inside muscles. Repeat 8 to 16 times.

Biceps (2)
Fronts of arms
Stand with your knees bent and your buttocks tucked under to protect your lower back.

Keeping your elbows into your waist and your shoulders down, slowly raise and lower dumb-bells with alternate arms. Repeat up to 30 times, depending on weights.

Press-ups (4)
This movement works your arms and chest.

Kneel on the floor with your ankles crossed. Keep your buttocks tucked under and your shoulders down.

Lean on to your hands. Walk forwards on them until they are aligned under your shoulders, pointing forwards.

Bend your arms, lowering your chest to the floor smoothly. Straighten your arms slowly (without locking your elbows) and repeat 8 to 16 times. *Note*: the closer your arms are to your knees the less weight you lift.

4

2

BACK STRENGTHENERS

Gently exercising your upper body and back instantly improves posture and poise – you will look better and feel great.

Our upper bodies are often weaker than we would like. This is because most of our everyday tasks require us to reach forwards (round or over a desk, typewriter or cooker for instance) so that the muscles on the upper back are constantly being stretched while the chest muscles in front often become over-tight. This imbalance not only draws the shoulders forwards, opening out the shoulder blades and rounding the upper back, but also narrows and drops your rib-cage so that you are slumped out of alignment.

The muscles that help you maintain lift in your upper body are in the upper back, working rather like a corset that laces up behind. Tighten the lacing and correct posture is regained – no more rounded shoulders and cramped rib-cage.

Exercise is the key to creating this change. Warm up properly before carrying out any of the exercises here (see page 122).

Skincare

The skin on your back is thicker than that of the face and contains more sebaceous (oil) glands than other areas of the body. Be sure to cleanse the skin here thoroughly, using a back brush, or ask your partner to apply a body scrub once a week.

However, if your skin is *already* spotty, avoid abrading it in these areas or you may spread the infection. Instead, apply topical lotions to dry out the spots and be careful not to pick at them or they may scar.

If your back needs the professional touch, try a 'back facial' in a beauty salon, which will include massage and deep cleansing.

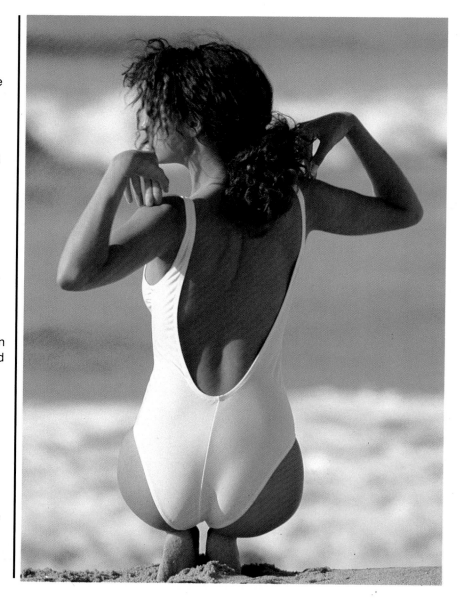

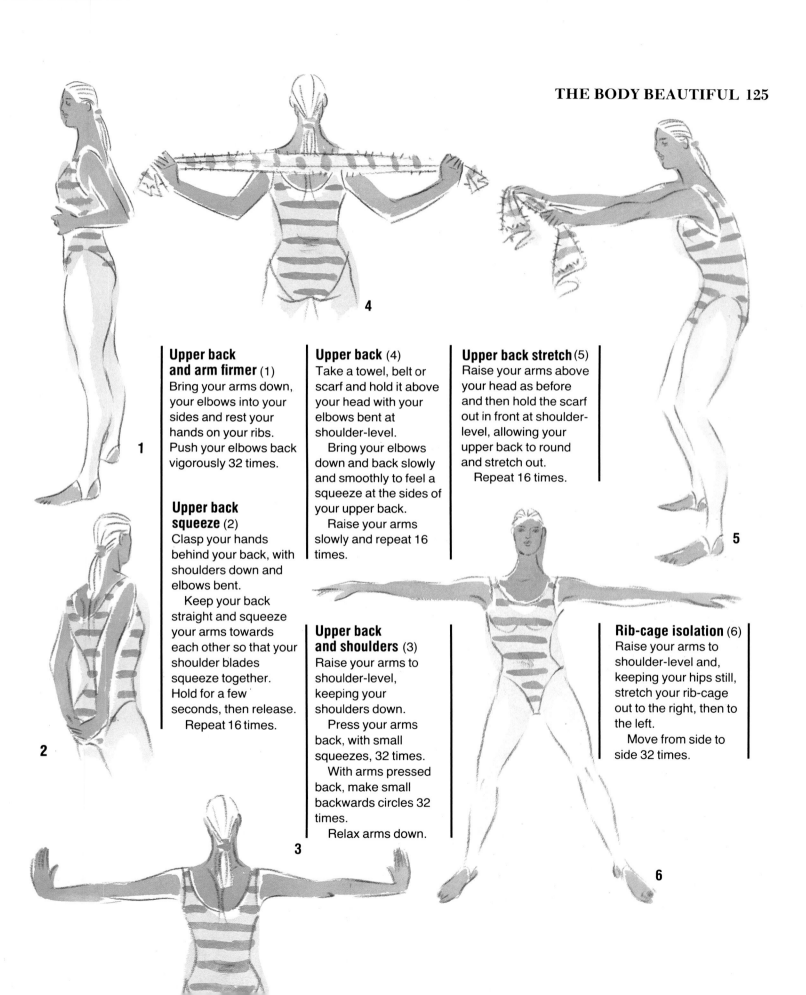

Upper back and arm firmer (1)

Bring your arms down, your elbows into your sides and rest your hands on your ribs. Push your elbows back vigorously 32 times.

Upper back squeeze (2)

Clasp your hands behind your back, with shoulders down and elbows bent.

Keep your back straight and squeeze your arms towards each other so that your shoulder blades squeeze together. Hold for a few seconds, then release.

Repeat 16 times.

Upper back (4)

Take a towel, belt or scarf and hold it above your head with your elbows bent at shoulder-level.

Bring your elbows down and back slowly and smoothly to feel a squeeze at the sides of your upper back.

Raise your arms slowly and repeat 16 times.

Upper back and shoulders (3)

Raise your arms to shoulder-level, keeping your shoulders down.

Press your arms back, with small squeezes, 32 times.

With arms pressed back, make small backwards circles 32 times.

Relax arms down.

Upper back stretch (5)

Raise your arms above your head as before and then hold the scarf out in front at shoulder-level, allowing your upper back to round and stretch out.

Repeat 16 times.

Rib-cage isolation (6)

Raise your arms to shoulder-level and, keeping your hips still, stretch your rib-cage out to the right, then to the left.

Move from side to side 32 times.

BUST BEAUTY

Make bustcare part of your beauty programme. Good skincare tactics and regular exercise will keep your breasts beautiful.

Care for your bust on a regular basis, with exercise and skincare, and you will be surprised what a difference this makes.

Follow our breast beauty plan and your bustline will always look its natural best.

Tips for beautifying your bust

• The breasts are supported by the fan of skin extending from the tip of the chin to just beneath the bust. It is therefore important to keep this skin firm and toned. Apply body lotion daily after bathing and never take baths that are too hot – very hot water breaks down the skin's connective tissues.

• Don't spray your decolleté with perfume – it will cause this delicate skin to dry.

• When sunbathing, always wear sunscreens on your chest and breasts and sunblock on your nipples.

• Correcting poor posture is an instant bustline improver (see page 124). Open out your chest by rolling your shoulders back.

• Exercise the chest muscles three times a week. Exercising the pectoral muscles that lie under the breasts, across the shoulders and upper arms gives the bust added lift. Exercise does not increase the size of the breasts as they do not contain any muscle.

• Crash diets are very bad news for bust-conscious women, leading to stretch marks and sagging.

• Choose a bra made from natural fibres that is not too tight (a very tight bra restricts circulation). Avoid wearing padded bras too often as they cause sweating, which is detrimental to the condition of the skin. Always, always wear a bra when exercising.

• It is essential that you check your breasts for any changes or lumps every month from puberty. Do this on the same day each month, a few days after your period, when changes in the feel and size of your bust due to fluctuating hormone levels will have normalized.

Position for exercises

Lie with two pillows under your head and upper back or on a thick exercise mat. Your elbows should be able to dip below chest-level.

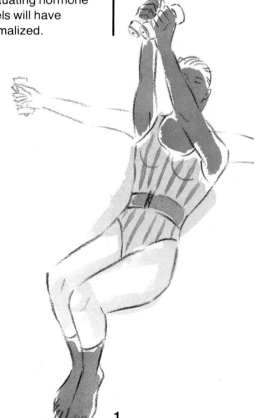

1

Use dumb-bells (see page 122 for weights).

Start with 10 repeats of each exercise and work up to 20 or 30, leaving a day between each workout. Keep your lower back pressed into the floor.

Chest builder (1)

With your hands lightly grasping the weights, extend your arms straight up, your palms facing each other.

Inhale and slowly pull your arms apart, slightly bending your elbows as you lower your arms smoothly towards the floor.

Exhale and bring your hands back together.

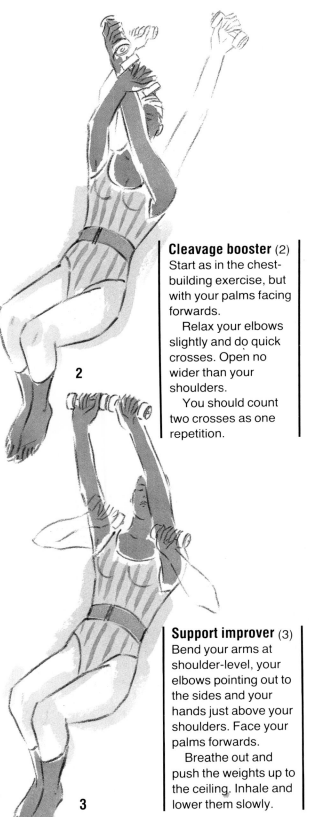

Cleavage booster (2)
Start as in the chest-building exercise, but with your palms facing forwards.

Relax your elbows slightly and do quick crosses. Open no wider than your shoulders.

You should count two crosses as one repetition.

Support improver (3)
Bend your arms at shoulder-level, your elbows pointing out to the sides and your hands just above your shoulders. Face your palms forwards.

Breathe out and push the weights up to the ceiling. Inhale and lower them slowly.

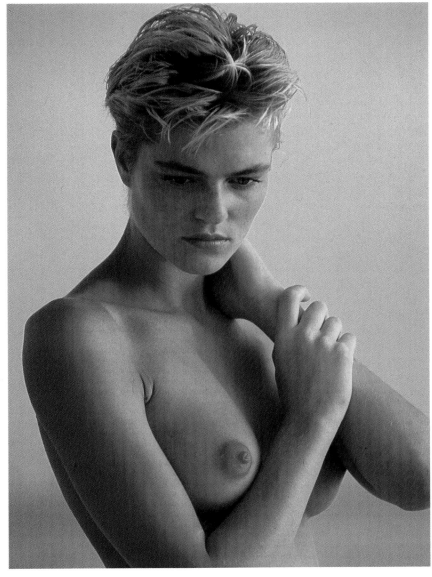

STOMACH AND WAIST FLATTENERS

Developing a stronger, flatter stomach calls for special exercises and a little determination, but we have made it as easy as possible.

Women are physically designed to have a slightly rounded abdomen. In addition, excess fat is readily deposited here.

A healthy, low-fat eating programme and toning exercises will help you redefine a flabby stomach.

• Doing abdominal exercises correctly calls for determination and a fair amount of hard work. The short cut to a flatter stomach is good technique. Done correctly, abdominal exercises are very effective and are definitely worth the effort! Do the exercises regularly and your stomach will be stronger, firmer and flatter.

Straight sit-ups, which are also known as curl-ups, aren't enough. You must also work the upper and lower abdominals and the bands of muscles at the sides. Your stomach muscles should always be pulled in before you add any resistance, and you must hold them in throughout the movement. If you do abdominal exercises with your stomach bulging (for bulging read *straining*), they will develop that way. You will no longer be holding the weight of your body with your abdominal muscles and muscles attached to your lower back will take over. So, if you start to strain you should stop.

• Body-conditioning classes are an excellent place to start if you haven't exercised for a while. The teacher will take you through the movements step-by-step, should check that you are doing them correctly and will motivate you.

• In the gym, most weight-training systems will include some exercises for the stomach area and you may find that simply having a bar to hold on to as you lie on a slanted exercise bench and bend and lower your legs will help you to grit your teeth and carry on!

At-home and salon treatments

You should be very gentle with your stomach: avoid using massage gloves and mitts in this area altogether.

In the salon, the Ionithermie treatment described on page 54 can be used from beneath the bust and is useful in reducing the size of the stomach to a small degree.

The exercises described here should, ideally, be done three times a week with a day's rest in between.

Stop exercising if you feel any strain in your lower back or if your stomach bulges and quivers. If you have a back problem, you should be

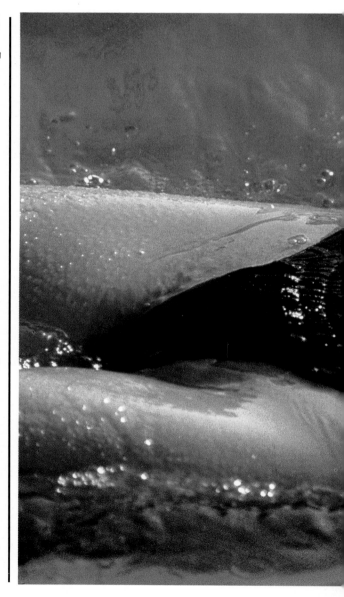

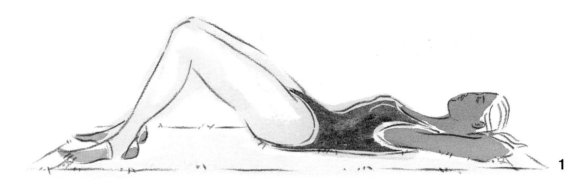

1

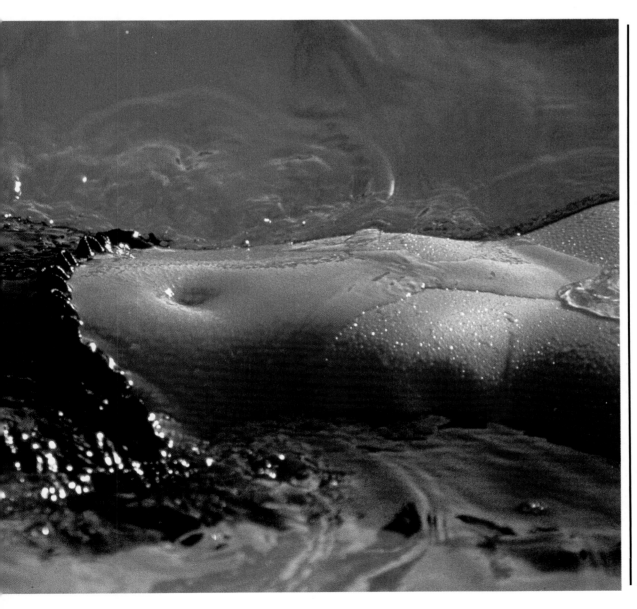

especially careful when doing stomach exercises. Begin with the first exercise, placing your legs over the seat of a chair, and add the others over a period of time, depending on your level of fitness.

Lie on an exercise mat or on two towels throughout the exercises.

Warm up
Walk briskly around the room for a few minutes before you begin.

Pelvic tilt (1)
Lie on your back with your feet flat on the floor, hip-width apart, knees bent.

Breathe out as you pull your lower stomach in hard and press the small of your back firmly to the floor, lifting your buttocks slightly.

Repeat this exercise 20 times.

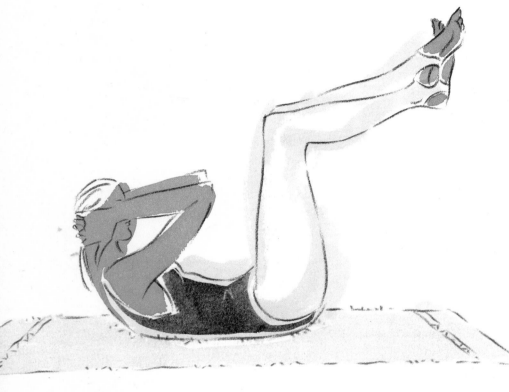

2

Upper abdominals (2)
Lie on your back with your feet off the floor and your legs bent at a right angle.

Pull your stomach muscles in so that your pelvis tilts and your lower back presses into the floor.

Cross your feet.

Place your hands by the sides of your head, elbows out.

Gently lift your shoulders from the floor and try to touch your elbows to your knees without moving your thighs.

Don't allow your legs to drop forwards (if they do, rest your legs over the seat of a chair).

Return to the start position and repeat 10 to 20 times.

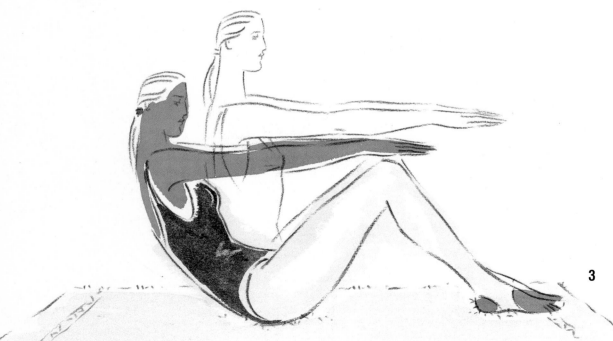

3

Total abdominals (3)
Sit with your knees bent, your feet flat on the floor and your arms straight out in front.

Be sure to keep your chin tipped down to your chest and stomach in as you *slowly* lower your upper body back towards the floor, rolling down through the spine and controlling the weight of your body with your stomach muscles. Finish when your shoulders touch the floor, keeping your head off the floor.

Return to the start position and repeat 5 to 10 times.

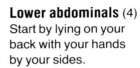

Lower abdominals (4)

Start by lying on your back with your hands by your sides.

Pull in your stomach muscles so that your pelvis tilts and your lower back presses into the floor.

Bend your knees into your chest and lift your legs up until they make a right angle with your upper body.

Cross your ankles.

Without pushing off the floor, lift your hips using your lower abdominals – your knees should come a little way towards your shoulders.

Then, lower your hips back to the floor and repeat 10 to 15 times.

Note: it can take time before you feel any effect in the correct areas, so persevere. You should feel the movement pulling in from the pubic bone and into the lower part of your stomach, but it should not be painful.

4

Upper abdominals and waist (5)

Start in the same position as for upper abdominals, but only bend one leg, leaving the other extended.

Twist your shoulders so that the opposite elbow points towards the raised knee. Reverse the legs and twist the other way.

Start slowly and gradually increase the speed, getting into a rhythm. Repeat 10 to 20 times.

Note: your straight leg adds the weight for the stomach muscles to resist against. Start with your legs fairly high for less weight. Make sure that you can hold in your stomach against the weight you're adding.

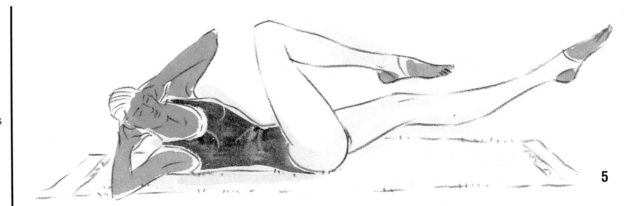

5

Muscle soother (6)

After performing stomach exercises, relax your muscles by lying on the floor and bringing your knees to your chest, keeping your lower back pressed into the floor. Clasp your hands over your knees.

Breathe in slowly and deeply several times.

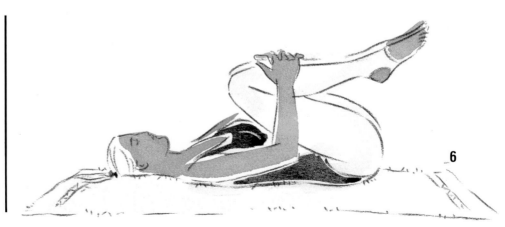

6

HIP, THIGH AND BOTTOM TONERS

Re-size your thighs, hone your hips and perk up your posterior with these on-the-spot exercises and firming treatments.

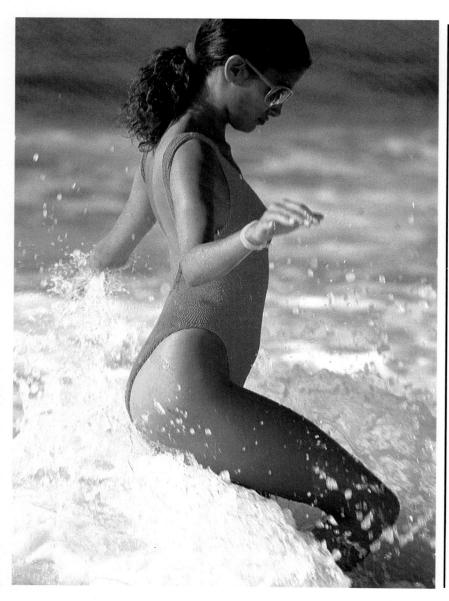

The hips, thighs and bottom are the number one problem area for the majority of women. The simple fact is that we are physiologically built to deposit fat around the hips and buttocks.

You can re-shape this body zone, however, by using the special toning and firming exercises described on the following pages.

WHAT IS CELLULITE?

This is the dimpled, 'orange peel' skin that often forms in puberty, when we increase our weight, and just before the menopause. Toxins, fluid and fat accumulate, weaken the tissues and prematurely age the structure of the skin. While hormonal changes are a prime cause, there are several other important contributing factors.

● Toxins are trapped in the area due to poor circulation. When fighting cellulite, you should eat a wholefood diet and drink plenty of water. Give up stimulants such as coffee, nicotine and alcohol that are heavily implicated in the formation of cellulite. Avoid salt, sugar and processed foods and limit the amount of fat, dairy produce and meat you eat.

● A sedentary life-style and wearing tight clothes such as jeans leads to poor circulation in the area. Stress can worsen the problem, tense muscles leading to restricted lymph drainage. Walk and swim as often as possible.

At-home treatments

Regular massage with a mitt and a body-contouring gel will boost the effects of the anti-cellulite tactics above. Don't rub too hard with a massage glove, however, or you may break small capillaries. Simply massaging with your hands helps too. Using your whole hand, gently squeeze the skin, moving it from one hand to the other. Use aromatherapy oils such as cypress and juniper to enhance the action. Remember that whenever you massage you should move towards your heart, in harmony with your circulation.

Dry skin brushing is another cellulite beater. By stimulating lymph drainage this deceptively simple treatment can have tremendous benefits for all-round health. It takes just a few minutes a day.

Before bathing or showering, use a brush made of very stiff, natural bristles to make circular movements all over the hip and thigh area. If you have time, use long, firm movements from your foot up to your knee, and then up to your thigh. Next, focus on your hips and buttocks. Use the brush very gently at first. If it is scratching your skin, soak it in warm water and then leave it to dry before using it again.

Salon treatments
There are a number of salon treatments that speed up the treatment of cellulite.
- Aromatherapists use special blends of essential oils to tackle the area, usually to great effect.
- Health spas and health farms offer a range of solutions from seaweed baths, which have a detoxifying and mild slimming effect, to hydrotherapy, where the aesthetician aims jets of sea-water at the flabby areas.
- G5 massage uses electrically-powered massage heads to improve circulation.
- Treatments such as Ionithermie are very effective at flushing out retained fluid and a reduction of several inches can be achieved over the whole area in one session.

Gels and creams containing active ingredients are applied to the skin, then clay is smoothed on and electrodes inserted in between the layers. Two types of current are then applied: faradic current to exercise the muscles passively – you feel fairly strong tingling and twitching sensations in your muscles – and galvanic current, which increases the absorption of the products. The inches will stay off if you eat healthily and take regular exercise.
- Lymphatic drainage treatments are becoming increasingly available. The lymph drainage circulation is the body's waste disposal system and it can often become sluggish due to a lack of exercise and other factors. One salon method uses inflatable rubber 'stockings' that are zipped on to the leg from ankle to thigh. As the stockings inflate, the pressure pushes the lymph around the body. In fact, this treatment has benefits for total body health.

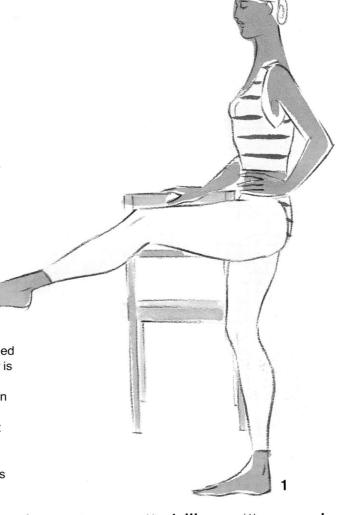

1

Warm up (1)
Use the back of a chair for balance.

Start with your outside foot behind you, then swing it forwards and back loosely, allowing your knee to bend.

Do this 16 times.

Then, using small movements, lift a little further up at each end of the swing 16 times.

Change to your left leg and repeat.

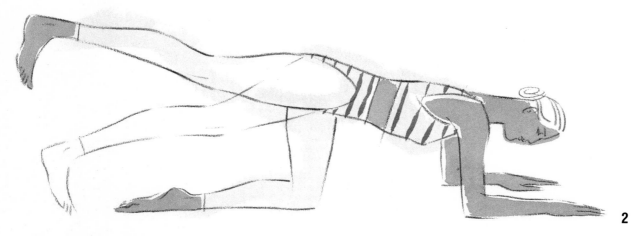

2

Backs of thighs and bottom

(2) Rest on your knees and forearms.

Hold your stomach in to keep your lower back straight and raise your right leg, keeping your leg straight and your foot flexed at a right-angle to your leg.

Touch the floor with your toe and then raise your leg using the back-of-thigh and buttock muscles.

Do this 16 times.

Then, using small movements, push up a little more at the top of the lift 16 times.

Repeat the exercise using your left leg.

(3) Lying on your front with your head resting on your arms, raise your right leg, keeping your right hip in contact with the floor.

Flex your foot and bend your knee so that your heel comes in towards your bottom.

Straighten your leg a little and repeat the movement 16 times.

Keep your leg bent and raise and lower your thigh 16 times.

Repeat the exercise using your left leg.

3

Inside thigh (4)

Roll on to your side.

Straighten your underneath leg and turn it out so that your knee faces forwards.

Bend your top leg and place your foot behind your lower leg.

Raise and lower your straight leg, using inside thigh muscles. Repeat 32 times.

Roll over and repeat using your other leg.

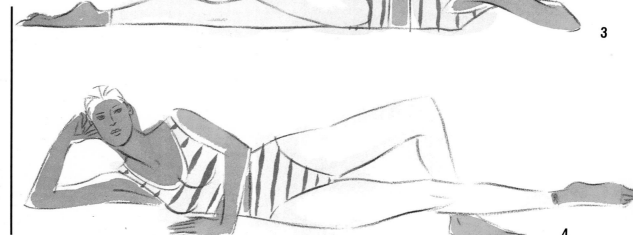

4

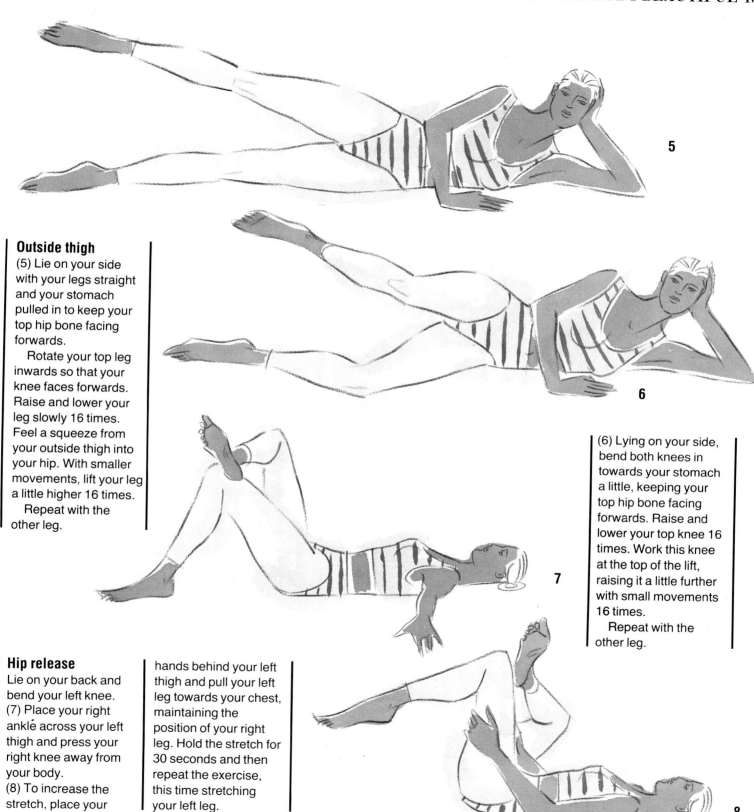

5

Outside thigh

(5) Lie on your side with your legs straight and your stomach pulled in to keep your top hip bone facing forwards.

Rotate your top leg inwards so that your knee faces forwards. Raise and lower your leg slowly 16 times. Feel a squeeze from your outside thigh into your hip. With smaller movements, lift your leg a little higher 16 times.

Repeat with the other leg.

6

(6) Lying on your side, bend both knees in towards your stomach a little, keeping your top hip bone facing forwards. Raise and lower your top knee 16 times. Work this knee at the top of the lift, raising it a little further with small movements 16 times.

Repeat with the other leg.

7

Hip release

Lie on your back and bend your left knee.
(7) Place your right ankle across your left thigh and press your right knee away from your body.
(8) To increase the stretch, place your hands behind your left thigh and pull your left leg towards your chest, maintaining the position of your right leg. Hold the stretch for 30 seconds and then repeat the exercise, this time stretching your left leg.

8

LEGS WORKOUT

Use these exercise and beauty secrets for lovelier legs – they are one of the easiest body areas to firm into shape.

Your basic leg shape is determined by your genes, though you can redefine it to a certain extent. Exercise will strengthen and sculpt, reduce flabbiness and ensure shapely calves and ankles.

As well as the exercises illustrated, make a conscious effort to use your legs more in day-to-day life: walk up and down stairs instead of using escalators and lifts, go on foot or cycle as often as possible. For the sports-minded, swimming, horse-riding, basketball and running are all great leg shapers.

If you are desk-bound all day the chances are that your legs will feel tired and ache and be prone to cramp. This is because sitting slows the circulation. Guard against this by stretching your legs every now and then and don't sit with them tightly crossed.

Try this quick circulation-boosting exercise, which will also firm your thighs and help flabby knees.
● Sit on a chair that supports your back.
● With your left foot flat on the floor, raise your right leg (so that it is parallel to the floor) until your knee locks.
● Bend your right leg a little way then straighten it again.
● Repeat 10 times and then do the same, stretching your left leg.

At-home and salon treatments

Remember that your legs are drier than other areas of your body, so moisturize them after every bath or shower.

Legs like to be exfoliated too, (see page 52), particularly the knee area. Try it once a week, it will only take a few minutes.

For salon cellulite beaters, see page 132.

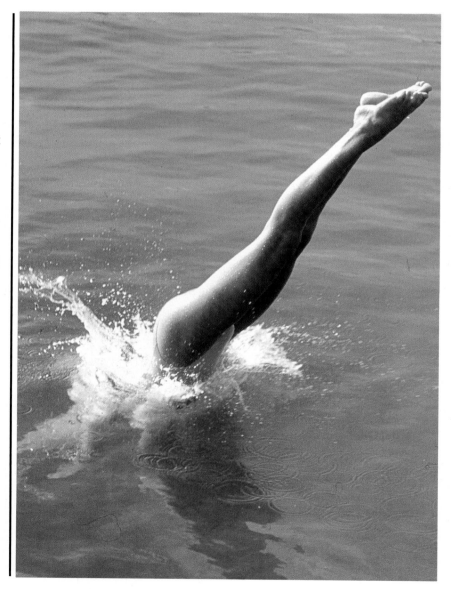

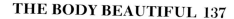

Front of thigh stretch (2)

This releases the muscles at the front of your thighs.

Lie face down. Bend your right foot towards your bottom, keeping your hips in contact with the floor. Hold your foot with your hands, and keep the position for 30 seconds. Repeat once with the other leg.

1

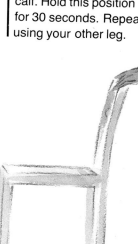

2

Front of thighs and knees (1)

Sit up straight with your left leg bent and your right leg straight out in front of you, with your knee facing up and your foot flexed. Raise and lower your leg smoothly 8 to 16 times. Repeat with your other leg, then do the front of thigh stretch.

Note: the muscles at the front of your thighs – the quadriceps – also support your knees, so by keeping them strong, you keep your knees stable.

Calves (3)

Using the back of a chair for support, place your feet together and tuck in your buttocks.

Raise and lower your heels smoothly. Repeat 16 to 32 times, then do the calf stretch.

Calf stretch (4)

Standing, slide your right leg back behind you without allowing your hips to twist. Press your heel to the floor and lean your weight forwards, keeping your body straight. Feel the stretch through your calf. Hold this position for 30 seconds. Repeat using your other leg.

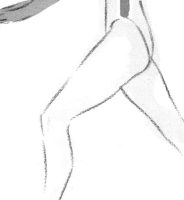

3

4

HAPPY HANDS, FABULOUS NAILS

Give your hands and nails the attention they deserve – don't neglect this important part of your total image.

A little regular care will keep your hands and nails looking their polished best. Follow the finger tips below and you'll have no excuse for untidy cuticles, brittle nails or dry hands.

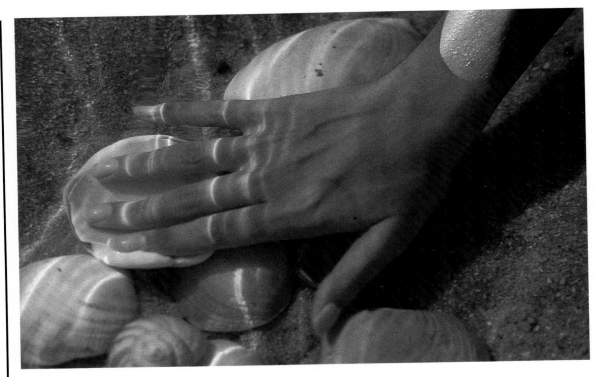

HANDCARE

● Do not plunge unprotected hands and nails into soapy water or household chemicals – wear rubber gloves!

● Apply handcream every time you wash your hands. Keep tubs of handcream beside the sink or basin.

● Remember to exfoliate the skin on the backs of your hands as well when you use a scrub on your body or face.

● Massage your hands with handcream whenever you have a few minutes to spare. Use the first finger and thumb of the opposite hand and work in small circles, moving from tips of fingers to wrist.

NAILCARE

● When you have a bath, push your cuticles back with your fingertips or a towel (use a light touch) as the warm water will have softened them.

● Nail nourishers are fast to apply and pay big beauty dividends, feeding the nail and surrounding skin with essential vitamins, oils and protein, helping the nails to grow.

● Manicure your nails fully approximately every 10 days, re-applying nail polish as necessary. Treat the cuticles very gently as they protect the growth centre of the nail. Never tear the skin or cut the cuticles.

● After removing nail polish you should wait a few minutes before filing. The nails may split if they aren't completely dry.

● Filing straight up against your nail can peel the tip: you should hold the emery board at a 45 degree angle under the free edge of the nail.

● The fastest way to prevent soft, weak nails from breaking is to apply hardener once or twice a week. It saves vulnerable nails and gives a high-shine finish.

● Brittle, peeling nails are caused by dryness. Massage handcream into nails frequently.

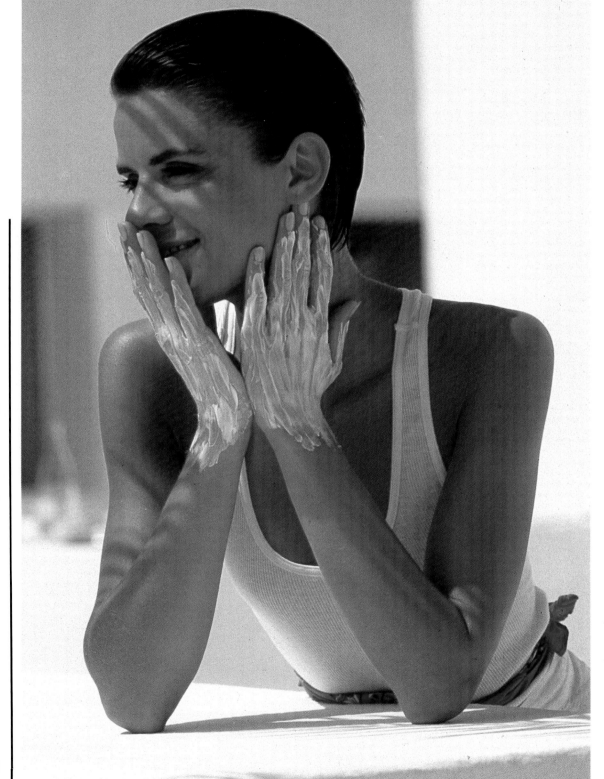

● Base coat is a good investment. Although it is formulated to help nail polish last longer, it also prevents bright colour from staining your nails.

● Use this quick removal tip if your nails are stained. Dip the tips in half a lemon for 15 seconds. The citric acid in the juice acts as a bleach.

Wash your hands afterwards so that the lemon juice does not dry your nails.

● Nail polish is another good nail protector. When applying polish, especially dark colours, apply two to three thin coats, rather than one thick coat for an even finish.

● Don't take polish right to the edges of the nails: it's quicker and neater to leave a thin strip down the side. Try this three-stroke method: apply the first stroke along the centre of the nail; then apply polish along both sides.

FEET FIRST

Pamper your feet as much as you can – not only will they look better but you'll ward off problems too.

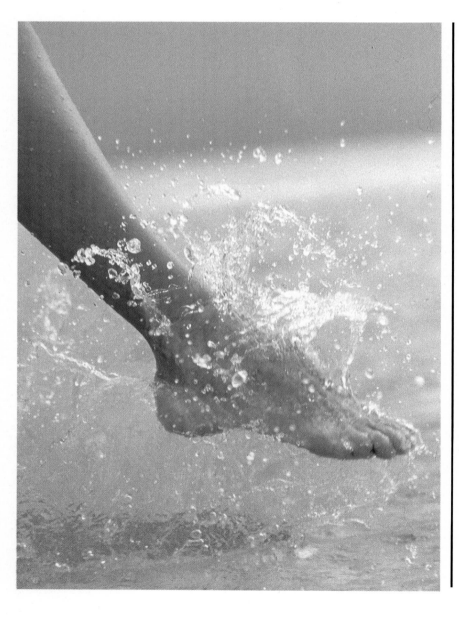

Feet are usually forgotten during a busy day, but often hurt most at the end of it. Looking after them is quick and easy.

FOOT WORKOUT

● Tired feet feel better fast with a massage. Use a refreshing cream or oil (with peppermint for instance) and work your thumbs in a circular motion starting at the ball of the foot, moving backwards towards your heel. Return to the toes, massaging each individually.

● Take the opportunity to walk barefoot whenever you can, allowing your feet free movement. Going barefoot in the sand is particularly good as it shapes the calves and ankles too.

● This exercise will strengthen your arches. Stand up straight with a tennis ball or rolling pin under one foot. Roll it backwards and forwards 10 times and then swap to the other foot and repeat.

● Stretch your feet out frequently, alternately flexing from the ankle and then pointing the toes.

● Circle your foot to the right eight times and then to the left eight times.

SHOE SENSE

The ideal shoe, allowing for toe shape, is 1.5 cm (½ in) longer than your foot. It should fit comfortably round the heel, over the instep and big toe. Leather is the best material, as it is permeable, allowing absorption of perspiration. A low, broad heel stresses the foot least. Sandals are good news for feet, too, as they don't restrict the toes and allow air to circulate.

Changing your shoes once or twice a day ensures that no one part of the foot has too much strain exerted on it.

Choosing shoes

During the day your feet swell. If you are choosing shoes, buy them in the afternoon to allow for this.

PERFECT PEDICURE·

Keep your feet looking good with a once weekly treatment. This do-it-yourself pedicure only takes about 10 to 15 minutes.

1 Remove old nail polish, then file or clip your toe-nails straight across.

2 Remove the cuticles with cuticle cream and a special implement — these can be found at the chemist.

3 Exfoliate the soles of your feet using water-dampened sea-salt.

4 Soak your feet for a few minutes in a warm foot bath, dry them thoroughly and follow with a massage as described in the foot workout above.

5 Before painting your nails, rub off any excess cream or oil, as it may cause the polish to slip.

6 Apply a base coat and two coats of colour for a long-lasting finish. If you haven't the time to allow the polish to dry naturally, use a quick-drying spray or run cold water over your nails.

Quick foot pacifiers for aching feet

● Kick off your shoes and lift your feet on to a desk or table or lie on your bed with your feet raised resting on two pillows.

● Wrap ice cubes in a flannel and rub over your feet up to your ankles. Dry each foot and then dab them with witchhazel.

● Soak your feet in a bowl of lukewarm water containing a foot spa solution.

● Apply a cooling foot lotion over your feet and legs, up to the knees.

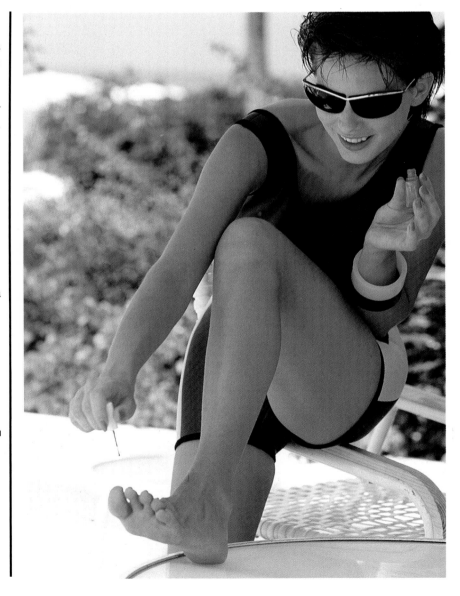

SMOOTH HAIR REMOVAL

Bothered by superfluous hair? Be a smooth operator and choose the best method for trouble-free hair removal.

Hair on the body is quite normal, yet cultural practices, fashion, hygiene and self-consciousness mean that hair removal is included in nearly every woman's beauty routine.

An alternative to removing hair completely on arms and upper legs is bleaching which can effectively disguise dark or thick hair. At-home kits are safe, if used correctly, but always do a patch test first in case of an allergic skin reaction.

SHAVING

Probably the most popular type of at-home hair removal, it cuts the hair down to the surface of the skin, removing some of the skin's outer layer.

Pain factor
Zero, unless you cut yourself.

Time factor
Takes a few minutes.

Regrowth
Starts to look and feel stubbly after a few days. Needs re-doing about twice a week to keep smooth. Hair grows back coarser.

Shaving tips
● To prevent irritation, use moisturizing shave cream and a razor with a comb guard.
● Use a special electric shaver for the sensitive bikini line.
● If you're off to the beach, shave the day before to allow the skin to recover – soreness can be triggered by chlorine, sunscreens and perspiration.

WAXING

This can be done both at home and in the salon, though salon waxing tends to be more effective.

Wax is usually heated and then pulled off in strips with paper or gauze against the direction of hair growth, pulling hair out from the follicle. Most salons use the 'cold' (in fact, warm) wax system. Hot waxing is less widely available, though more effective.

Pain factor
Ouch! Stings, but it's quick. You get used to it. Many people report that hot waxing is more painful than cold.

Time factor
A half-leg wax (both legs, knees to ankles) takes about 10 minutes.

Regrowth
Anything from three to six weeks depending on your rate of hair growth. Hairs grow back finer after repeated treatments.

Wax fax
● Hair has to be long enough to be covered by the wax. If it's too short, it either won't come out or will be removed patchily to the surface only, with disappointing results.
● Don't wax broken or irritated skin.
● To minimize irritation, the skin should be pulled taut before stripping. Afterwards little pimples may break out, but they generally subside after a few days. To avoid further irritation, for the next 24 hours avoid the sun, very hot showers, products containing alcohol or fragrance, deodorant if the underarms have been waxed and strenuous activity which will cause perspiration.
● If you find you get ingrowing hairs after waxing, use an exfoliator to help them grow correctly.
● Waxing regularly is the best plan.

SUGARING

This is a sugar-and-water putty, applied to a small area at a time and pulled off against the hair growth. It is well known in the Middle East and increasingly available in salons elsewhere.

Pain factor
Marginally less painful than waxing.

Time factor
Half-leg sugaring takes about 45 minutes.

Regrowth
Four to six weeks depending on the rate of hair growth. Hair grows back slower and finer with successive treatments.

Sugaring savvy
● Sugaring is less expensive than waxing, but it's harder to find a salon that does it.
● Use the same after-care tips as for waxing.

DEPILATORY CREAMS

These dissolve the hair to just below the surface of the skin.

Pain factor

Zero, unless you experience an allergy. It is important, therefore, to do a patch test 24 hours beforehand.

Time factor

About 20 minutes.

Regrowth

Depilation will be necessary again after a week or so.

Depilatory pros and cons

Depilatory creams are quick and effective but fairly messy to use and often smell unpleasant.

ELECTROLYSIS

This is the only permanent solution to unwanted hair, though hormonal changes during the life cycle can cause new growth.

Electrolysis involves inserting a needle (check your salon uses disposable ones) into the follicle and destroying the hair with heat generated by an electric current.

Pain factor

A short and sharp wince. Women always seem more sensitive just before or during menstruation.

Time factor

5 minutes to half an hour depending on the area treated and your pain threshold. As hairs must be caught during an active cycle it can take months to eradicate the hairs completely.

Regrowth

Very slow during treatment. Once treatment is finished, negligible.

Electrolysis pros and cons

● You need to be dedicated to undergo the treatment – it's an effective, but very lengthy process.
● It can become expensive, depending on the area and strength of hair growth being treated. It is not, for example, economically viable to have your legs treated in this manner.
● DON'T use an at-home kit – you could scar yourself permanently.
● DON'T schedule your appointment just before a meeting or going out if you are having electrolysis on the face, as there will be a little puffiness and redness afterwards, although this goes after a few hours.
● Electrolysis is the only method you should use on facial hair. If you don't want to go under the needle, though, bleach it.

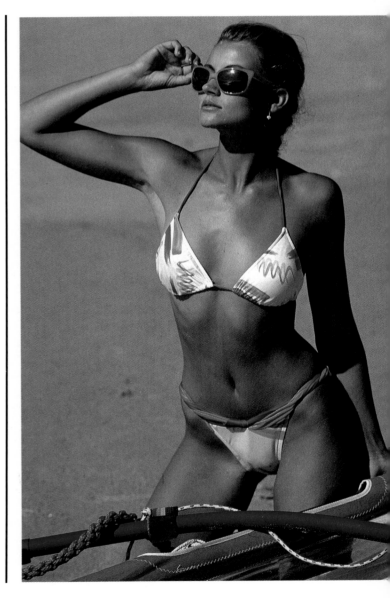

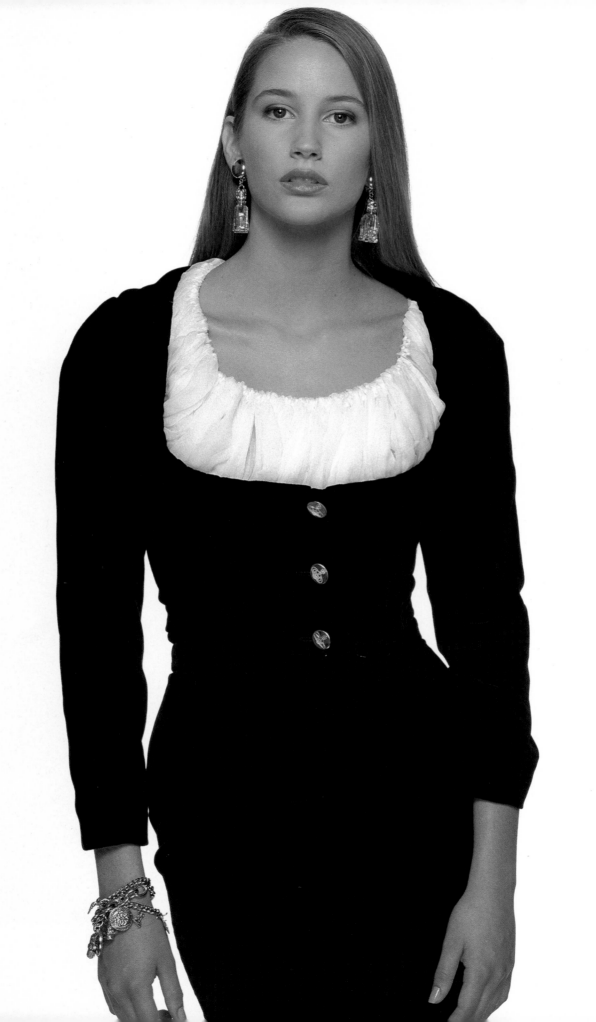

CLOTHES CONFIDENCE

We all want to present a well-groomed, stylish image to others, but it can be difficult to know where to start. The following pages are designed to give you ideas and helpful hints about clothes, colours and details which will help you to build a successful wardrobe and develop clothes confidence of your own.

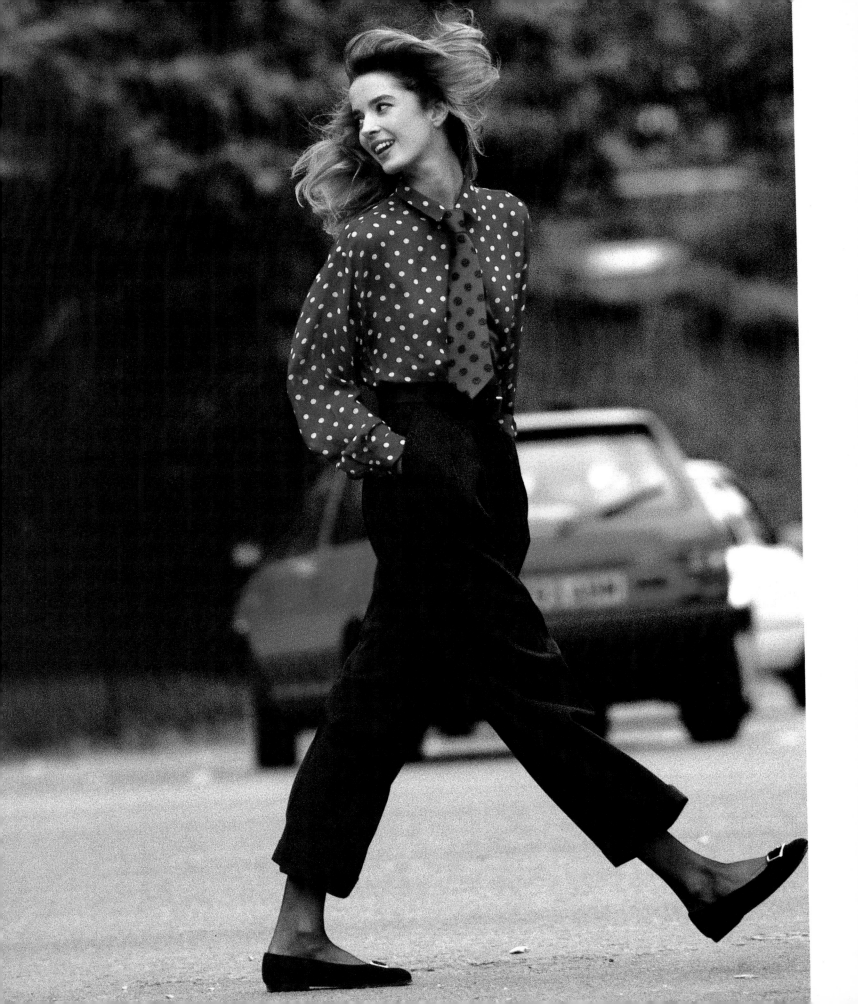

SHARPENING YOUR IMAGE

Clothes play a vital role in shaping other people's opinions of us. We'll help to ensure that you always make the right purchase.

The image we present to others through our clothes is remarkably important. The clothes and accessories we wear send implicit messages about our occupation and lifestyle, our emotions and interests.

We can use clothes as a dual-purpose confidence trick. Studies have shown that we react more favourably to people whose appearance appeals to us. By dressing with a sense of style, we are helping to ensure that others respond positively towards us. It is also true to say that when we look good, we feel better about ourselves, we feel more confident and capable and this is apparent to those around us.

A well-thought-out, though not necessarily extensive or expensive, wardrobe is all you need to carry you through. The secret of style is to select clothes that reflect your personality and fulfil as many as possible of the criteria below.

Confidence tricks

● Good quality fabric and cleverly cut clothes are worth investing in. Never buy anything that is too tight or that you don't feel really good in.
● Decide which colours you love to wear and aim to co-ordinate your wardrobe so that you increase the versatility of your purchases.

● Accessories are essential details. Look for well-designed classic scarves, belts and bags which will last for years and increase the impact of every outfit.
● Take notice of the details of a garment when buying: check the standard of the stitching on jackets and shirts. Consider changing the buttons if the ones on the suit or jacket let down an otherwise stylish garment.
● Be guided by the current fashion trends but never be a slave to them. Always remain faithful to your *own* sense of style.
● Try to avoid impulse buying. These purchases invariably end up at the back of your cupboard. If you like to shop at the sales, make time to try clothes on properly, and go away and think about an outfit if you're the least bit unsure about it.
● Consider the potential 'cost per wearing' of everything you wish to buy. If you only wear a dress once or twice the cost per wearing is probably going to be very high, although you may think it is worth it for a very special occasion.
● Whenever you're unsure about whether or not to add another bracelet, sweep on a scarf or add the hat, it is usually best to leave the article in question in the wardrobe. The chances are you'll feel more comfortable when dressed subtly.

● Look after your clothes! Everything in your wardrobe should be clean, carefully pressed and have been checked to ensure that no mending is required. It is especially useful to go through your wardrobe at the change of seasons before you put your winter or summer clothes away for a few months. Hang or fold your clothes at the end of the day.

Start investigating your clothes cupboard now. Be ruthless and give away all those items you haven't worn for years. Remember that clothes should be a pleasure to wear and aim to put your own individual stamp of style on every outfit.

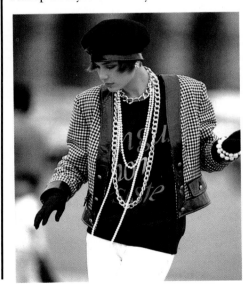

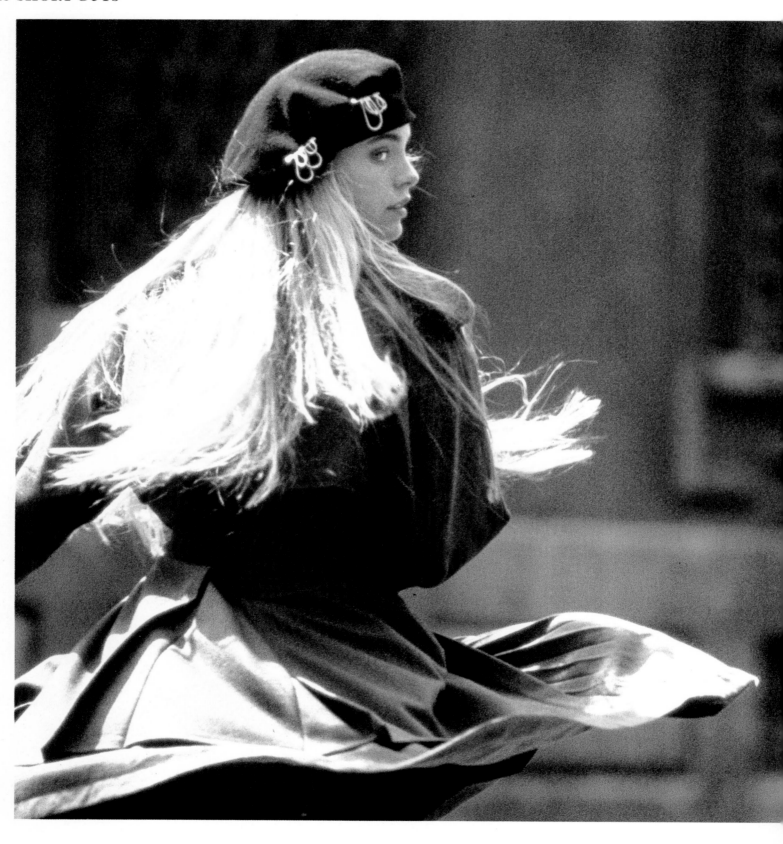

CLASSIC COATS

A coat can be the most difficult garment to buy – look for pure, natural cloths and well-designed details.

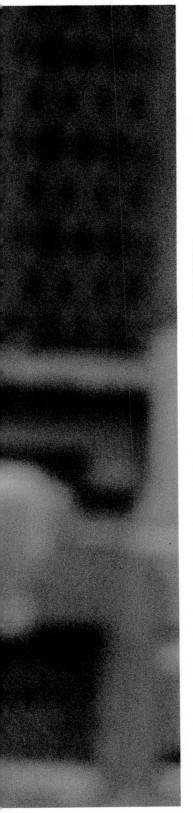

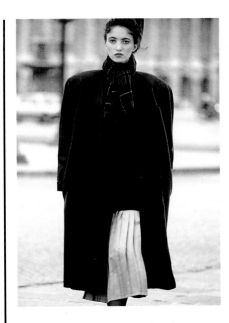

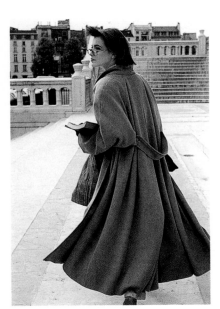

Cashmere, wool, camel . . . beautiful fabrics are part of the pleasure of owning a beautiful coat. A coat is probably the largest investment you will make for your wardrobe. It is worth spending as much as you can afford from your clothes budget in order to ensure a generous cut and the look of luxury that will last you at least several seasons, possibly many years.

The coat you choose will be influenced by the climate you live and work in. In temperate climes a lined raincoat may suffice, but if you travel or live in cold-weather countries you'll need a much heavier, warmer style.

There are several classic coat designs to choose from: trenchcoats with storm flaps and military-style epaulettes; Russian-influenced coats with fitted bodices, embroidered or fur-trimmed, and full skirts; mannish single-breasted overcoats with raglan sleeves; tailored double-breasted coats, shorter A-line coats which finish above or at the knee. Fake fur coats are a fun option.

When trying on a coat, try one or even two sizes larger than the size you would usually buy. You will find the bigger sizes tend to hang better – and will enable you to wear lots of layers underneath.

Neutral colours, especially taupe and camel which work with navy, black and brown, are often the most reliable choice for a coat that may have to cover up a wide variety of colours. Add extra colour with bright mufflers, hats and gloves.

Main picture
A short and swingy gaberdine raincoat is held in with a belt. Belted coats tend to be more flattering on tall people than short.
Above, left This collarless coat, cut straight from a broad shoulder line, is good for milder weather.
Above, right A long, full coat with raglan sleeves and a half-belt across the back is the classic cover-up.

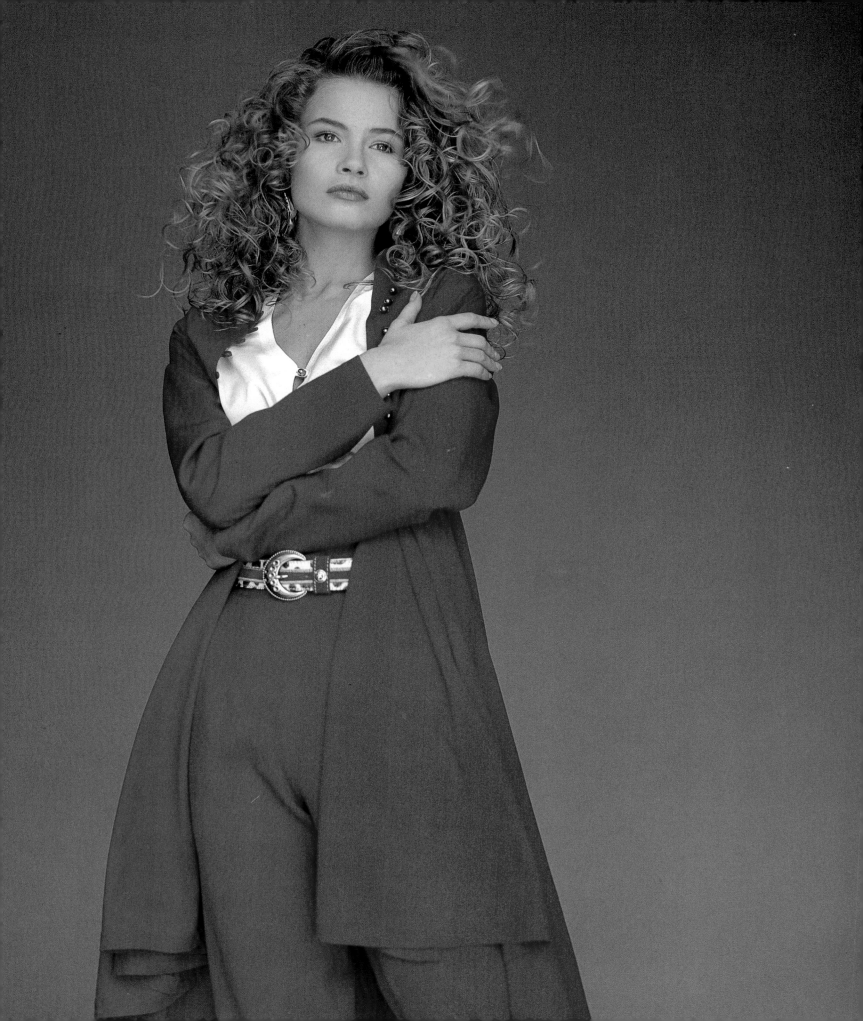

SEEING RED

Vibrant and confident, red is one of the new classic colours. Whether you want to look chic and sophisticated or sharp and trendy, it's guaranteed to get you noticed.

Red is a colour to be worn with confidence – unfortunately, too many women shy away from it, believing that as it's such a strong colour it won't suit them. While a completely red outfit can look overpowering on some people, touches of red, such as gloves, belts, bags or shawls, will always look smart and stylish.

There are plenty of reds to choose from, with either blue or orange undertones. It is a versatile colour choice, as it works with other primary or bright shades and instantly lifts grey, white and black. It looks fabulous with denim too.

Main picture An elegant trouser suit with swingy A-line coat jacket looks sophisticated, yet lively. The white top brightens the face and emphasizes the red. An unusual belt breaks up the block of colour.

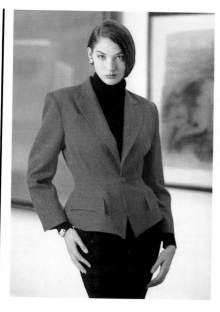

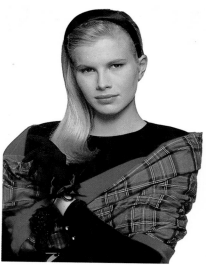

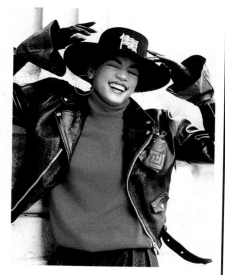

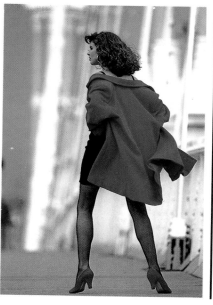

Far left, top A tailored orange-red jacket sets off a plain dress to perfection. The look is simple and streamlined, an excellent working outfit that retains a degree of glamour.

Left, top A pure cashmere sweater is a classic investment you'll never tire of. Team it with fun accessories and a leather jacket for a modern twist, or wear it with smart suits as an accent of colour.

Far left, below This traditional red tartan shawl instantly livens up a demure dress. It would also add style and warmth thrown over a plain coat.

Left, below A short, bright red coat will keep you warm and your spirits high on chilly days. This one is sophisticated enough to wear over a short cocktail dress. It could also be dressed down and worn with your favourite jeans.

NEW KNITS

Find your perfect jumper – from plain to patterned, warm and chunky to soft and close-fitting, there's something for everyone.

A soft knit with a round neck and long fitted sleeves is the traditional classic jumper. It looks good with trousers and skirts and can be used to brighten up a plain suit if it's in a vibrant colour. It is also easy to dress up with a scarf and jewellery.

There are plenty of variations on the jumper themes – different cuts and necklines, styles of knit and patterns. Arran, Shetland and Fair Isle sweaters are warm and casual but difficult to wear with anything else over the top as they are so bulky. If you like to wear a jumper under a jacket, thick, loose-fitting sleeves will be uncomfortable and spoil the line of the jacket. Wear a thermal vest or T-shirt under a thin knit if it's extra warmth you are after. Natural fibres usually feel more comfortable next to the skin than synthetic fibres. Cotton and cotton mixes are the ideal choice for warmer weather.

Look out for any jumpers with collar detail, such as lace and embroidery around the neck.

Jumpers should always be washed by hand and laid out flat to dry to keep their shape.

Below, left A Fair Isle knit works well as part of a country look and can be worn with other patterned clothes.

Below, centre A soft, long cardigan of lilac-tinted grey looks relaxed over lambswool leggings.

Below, right Give woollies shape by belting them.

Right Enveloping and warm, a traditional cream fisherman's sweater is brought up to date with contemporary stitching.

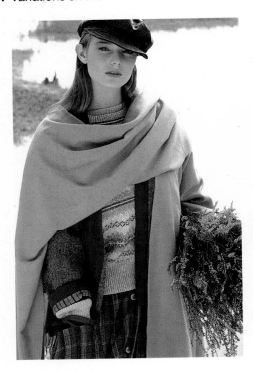

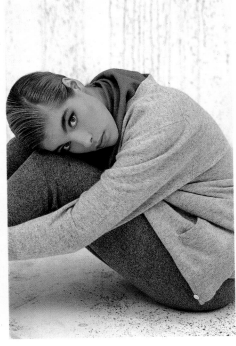

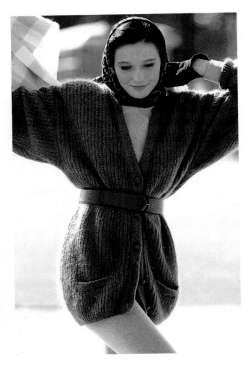

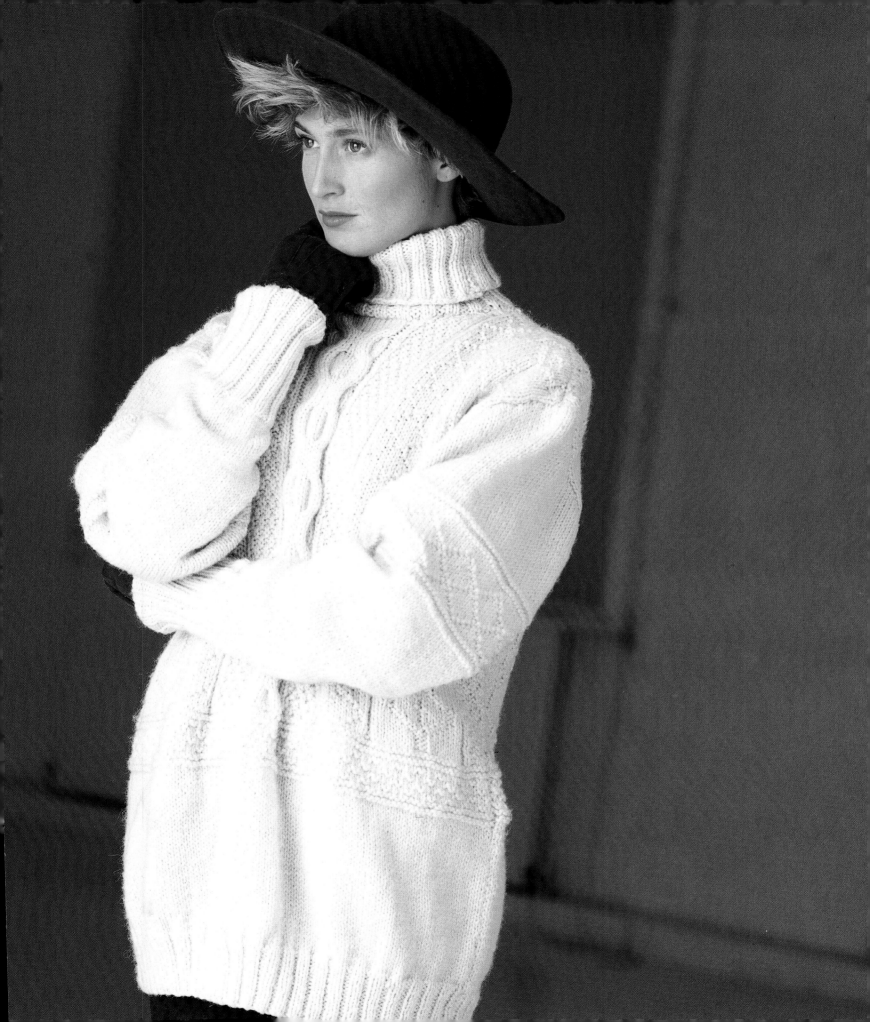

MOVING INTO NEUTRAL

These are the colours that clever women build their wardrobes around: neutral shades that can be mixed together to create slick city looks.

The neutrals are colours that never go out of style: there's black, of course, take-you-anywhere navy, and grey in every shade, from deepest charcoal to slate to palest silver grey. Then there are the brown hues: from rich, peat brown to taupe and stone, through to beige and cream. Neutrals suit everyone and always look upmarket.

By ensuring that key garments are cut to classic shapes in good cloth and neutral shades, you will have clothes that you'll always feel well-dressed in. Pivotal items to buy in neutral shades include raincoats, tailored trousers, bags, belts and shoes. Don't forget, though, that pale shoes, such as beige and cream shades, will make your feet look longer. Stick to the darker neutrals if you want to make your feet look smaller.

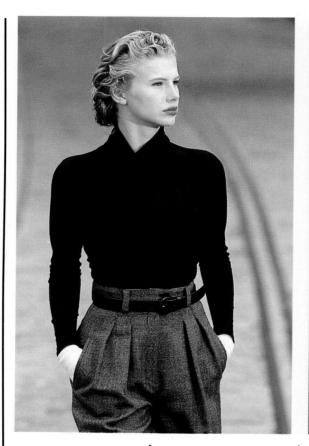

Above A simple cotton lycra, black body-skimming wrap top is teamed with pleat-front grey wool pants. The effect is stark and stylish. These garments would look fabulous in any of the neutrals. Imagine, for example, the same shapes but with a cream top and fawn trousers, or stone with charcoal grey. The secret of success is to mix and match the colours in simple, smart shapes.

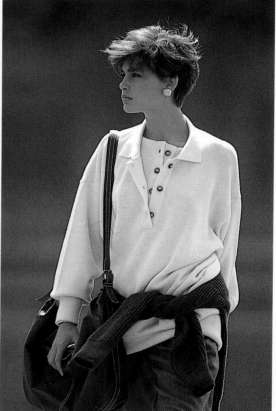

Above A clever combination of a slash-neck top in cream under a colour-matched long, loose tunic sweater looks effortless and modern. The dark plummy-grey ribbed sweater and slightly lighter grey trousers tone in with the cream and the brown leather-trimmed saddle bag. Finish the outfit with a pair of plain brown or two-tone brogues.

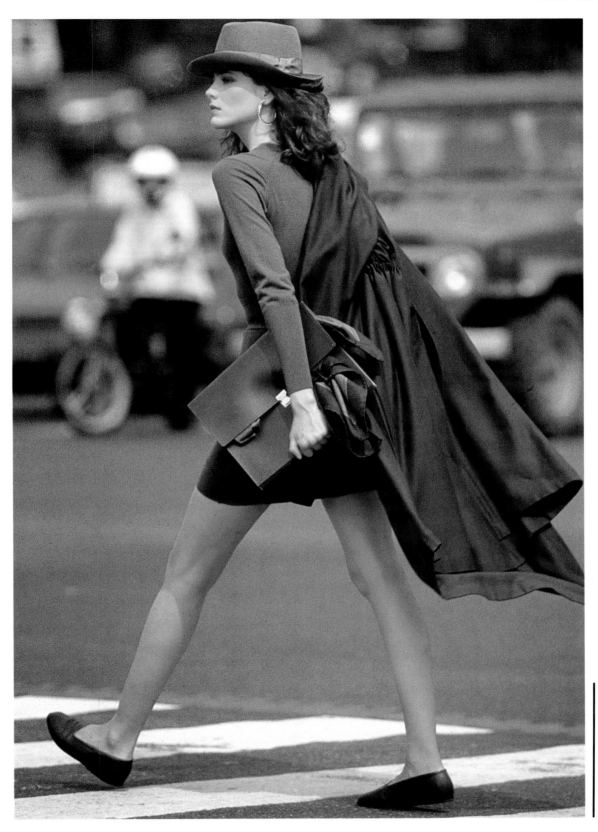

Left Young and city-smart, this look features a slate grey jersey top, navy short skirt plus toning silk scarf tied to the case. Co-ordinated accessories say 'this woman means business'.

EASY IN DENIM

Hardwearing and versatile, denim is a fabric that looks good whatever your age and never goes out of style.

Denim is made to last. It's also comfortable, easy to clean and adaptable. It is one of the best-known fabrics in the world and hugely popular, particularly as jeans – most people own at least one pair at some stage of their lives. Normally denim fades with washing. There are also specially treated styles; stone or milk washes, for instance, which give a light marbled effect, and bleaches which make denim very pale blue. Black denim is also widely available. Jeans come in a variety of cuts and fits, and styles go in and out of fashion; the best advice is to buy a pair that you feel comfortable in and personally like the look of. Although they will probably last for years, don't discard them when they start to look tired or when you buy another pair. Simply chop off the legs and wear them on holiday

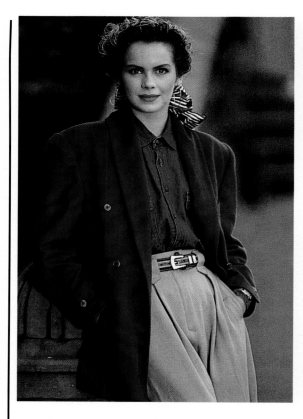

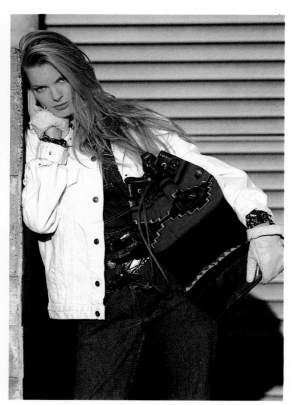

or at the weekend, teamed with a cropped top or baggy T-shirt.

As well as jeans, denim is also used for skirts, shirts and jackets – all easy-to-wear garments. So too are clothes in the denim look-alike chambray, which is softer to the touch. Classic blue denim looks excellent with a variety of other coloured items from brights to neutrals and black and white. It's very adaptable and, with the right accessories, can be dressed up or down.

Above, left A dark denim shirt looks smart with tailored trousers and a long jacket. For a more casual look try leaving the shirt unbuttoned and knot the ends together around your waist. *Above right* Denim dungarees look fun with long- or short-sleeved T-shirts (try stripes) or simple collared shirts. In this outfit, the dungarees are made part of an ethnic look with the addition of several big-buckled belts and a colourfully patterned duffle bag.

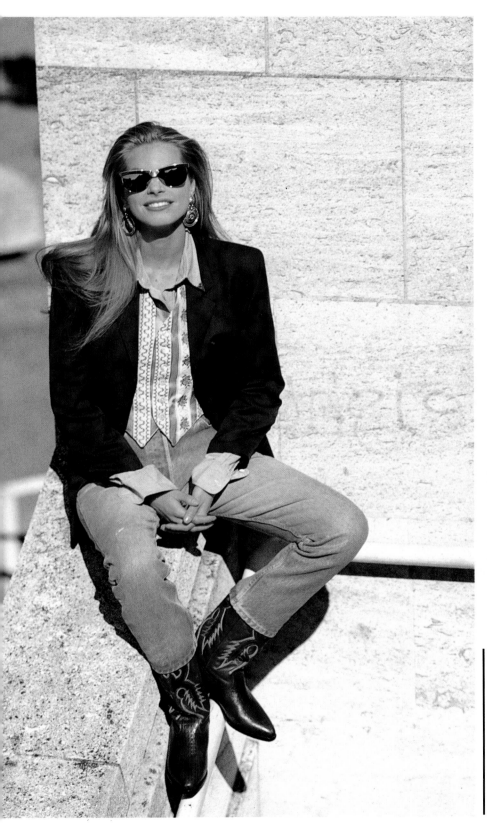

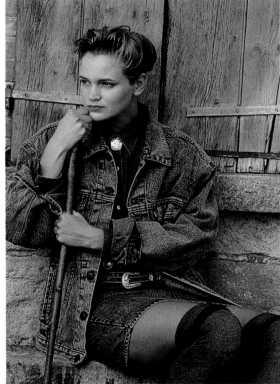

Left Western styling for urban life – classic faded jeans look their best with cowboy boots. A chambray shirt is teamed with a waistcoat and jacket to add interest above the waist. Chunky silver ear-rings are just right as accessories – too much would clutter the simple look.

Above Denim of differing shades can mix well together, but add some well-placed accessories. Black or brown buckled belts always look good with denim as does metallic jewellery.

CONTRASTING MOODS

Create style with impact in chic black and white – a truly sophisticated combination.

Black and white always look dramatic. The contrast of crisp white against sombre black looks expensive and also draws attention. Only a few can wear this combination without accessories though. It is definitely improved with the addition of jewellery and a bright scarf or gloves.

Both black and white carry strong associations. Black is linked to mourning, old age in Mediterranean countries, and also youth rebellion. It has certainly been adopted by the fashion world as the essential colour. Practically it is useful,

as it doesn't show marks as quickly as other colours. White is a symbol of purity and innocence. It always looks fresh and appealing. Worn close to the face, it brightens the complexion. Its only disadvantage is that it looks dirty quickly.

It's a sensible investment to incorporate a few black and white items into your basic wardrobe to mix and match with each other and with your other clothes. Stylish essentials are a white shirt, a pair of black tailored trousers for

winter and lighter ones for summer, a classic black skirt and a simple, little black dress for day-into-evening wear. Several pairs of leggings in both colours can be very useful to wear with long jackets, tops and big jumpers.

Left A white 'body' (an all-in-one leotard-like garment) is worn underneath a drop-necked jacket. The clothes are balanced with sizeable silver ear-rings and a precise, strong make-up. Without these details, the black and

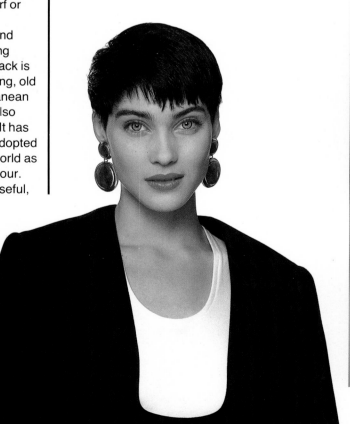

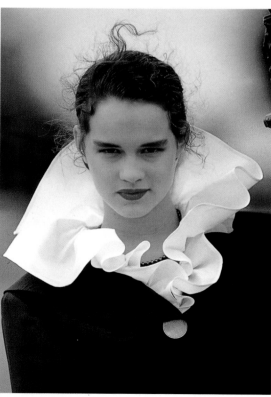

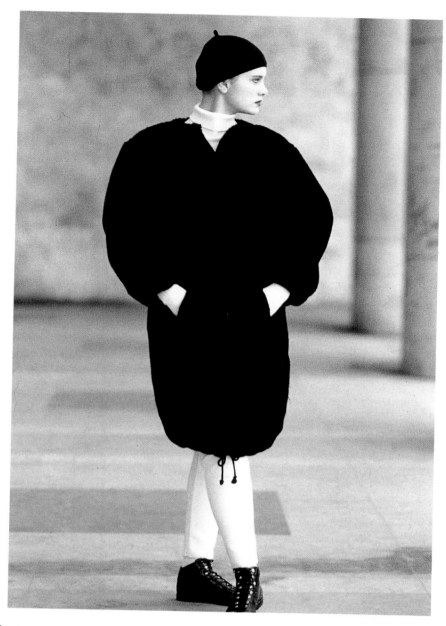

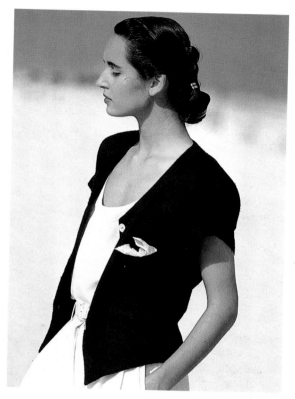

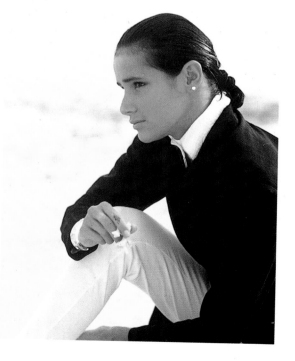

white would be too harsh, making the wearer look washed-out in comparison. *Left* A pure white ruffled collar focuses attention on the face. To keep the proportions correct, hair should be swept up as shown or kept short and neat.

Above Black and white for winter warmth – white leggings and a polo-neck jumper are topped with a padded black coat, given shape with a drawstring at the hem. Balance is kept with flat, black boots. *Above right* A white silk singlet gives an easy, simple feel underneath a shaped, cotton shirt.

Right Smarten up cotton leggings with a long black linen jacket and a white stand collar to add interest at the neck. Jewellery is minimal and hair sleeked back for a polished appearance.

SENSATIONAL SCARVES

Build up a collection of scarves and you instantly add many permutations to your wardrobe.

Originally worn chiefly by aristocrats, scarves are now a universal accessory. A designer scarf is a gilt-edged investment, giving the simplest outfit designer chic.

Look out for striking colour mixes and unusual designs. Floral and paisley patterns are classics, jungle prints look witty and lace makes a striking contrast set against a mannish tailored suit. Primary splashes of colour brighten the darkest-looking clothes in a flash.

There are myriad ways to wear scarves.
● Tied at the neck, a scarf can be simply knotted, worn as a bow over a stand-collared shirt, or gathered into an elaborate cockade.
● Smaller squares and rectangles can be tied in the hair: make a low ponytail and tie a scarf length just below the nape of the neck.
● Fold a scarf into a rectangle and make a headband, tying the ends in a soft knot on top, or wrap it around a chignon.
● Large scarves, shawls and wraps can lead another life worn as sashes around the waist and tied as tops.

Below Beautifully co-ordinated both in colours and proportions, classic grey flannel trousers are worn with a coffee-coloured shirt and cream wool cardigan. Note the different way of wearing a cardigan – unbuttoned and wrapped. The classic designer scarf is worn high on the neck and loosely knotted, the shades picking up and complementing colours in the clothing.

Below Clean shapes in black and white – a neat, above-the-knee skirt and a jacket shaped into the waist are given extra visual appeal with the addition of a patterned, red scarf.

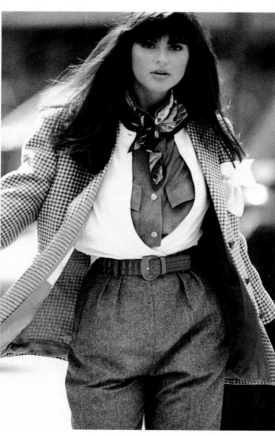

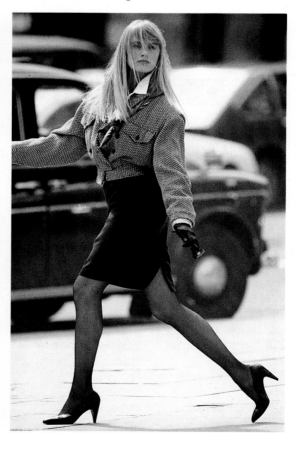

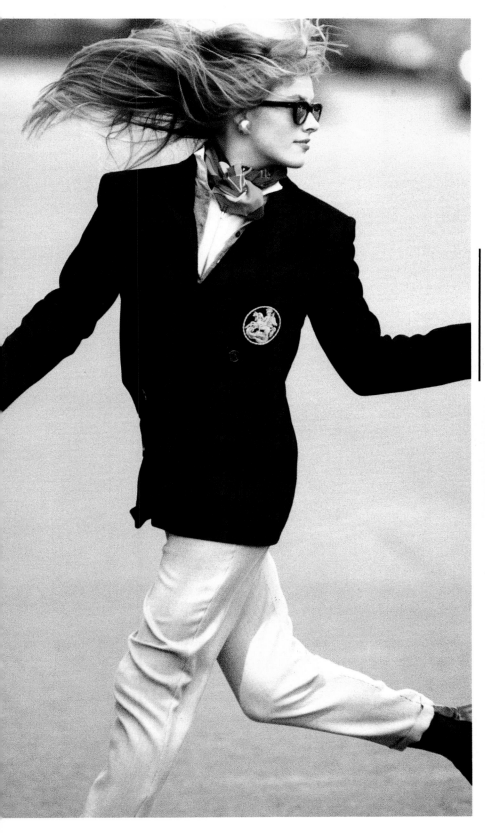

Left In a Deauville-inspired, smart, easy-to-wear outfit, tapered trousers are topped with a fresh white shirt, nautical blazer and a brilliantly-coloured scarf tied cravat-style at the neck.

Below Simple chic — a long, finely striped cotton voile scarf, is draped softly around the revers of a double-breasted cardigan. Pin the scarf in place with a brooch or two.

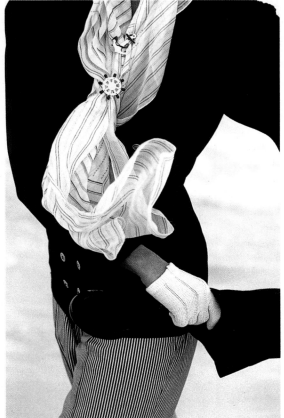

TAILOR-MADE

Polish up your image with impeccably-cut, tailored clothes.
They're working-style essentials!

Tailored clothes, with their air of formality, are a great choice for the working woman. Structured styles look best in quality fabrics such as wool. Always check that tailored garments are lined, they'll look and fit better, as well as lasting longer.

A good tailored jacket is the lynchpin of your wardrobe and it's worth going for the best you can afford, as quality will last you for several years, thus proving cost-effective in the long term. As a general rule, stick to more classic colours: good bets are black or navy for the winter and cream or cherry red for the summer. A tailored jacket can be very versatile, looking great with jeans for weekend wear as well as work-smart.

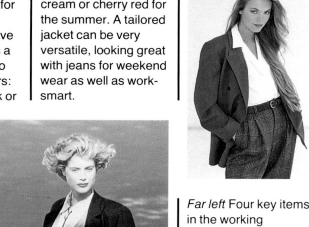

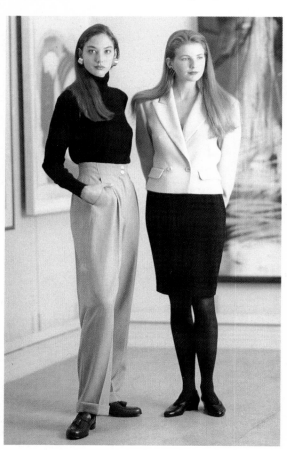

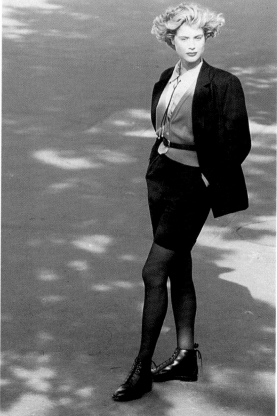

Far left Four key items in the working wardrobe: fawn, mannish pleated trousers, a wool and cashmere black polo-neck, a softly tailored jacket and a timeless knee-length black skirt.
Left Layer up under a smart black jacket with a belted cardigan and pastel pink shirt. Add an unexpected accessory like a bootlace tie for a witty touch.
Above Mix checked trousers with a plain jacket for a relaxed yet smart combination.
Right Tailoring can mean dressed to kill!

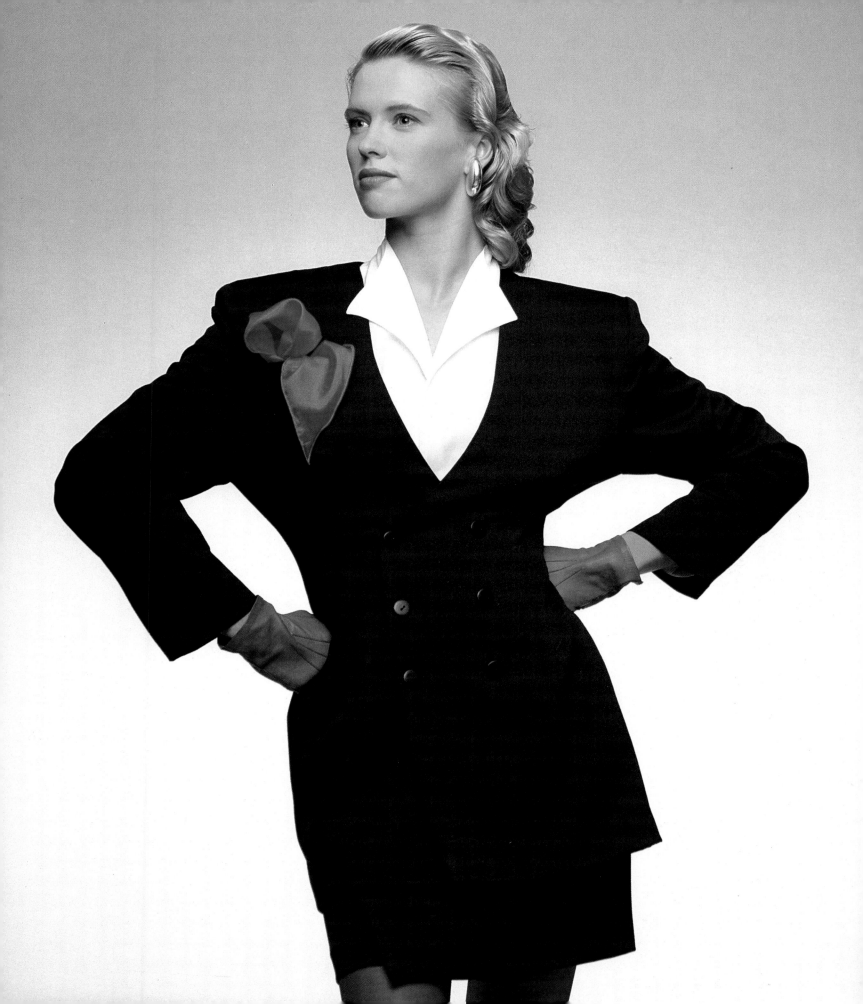

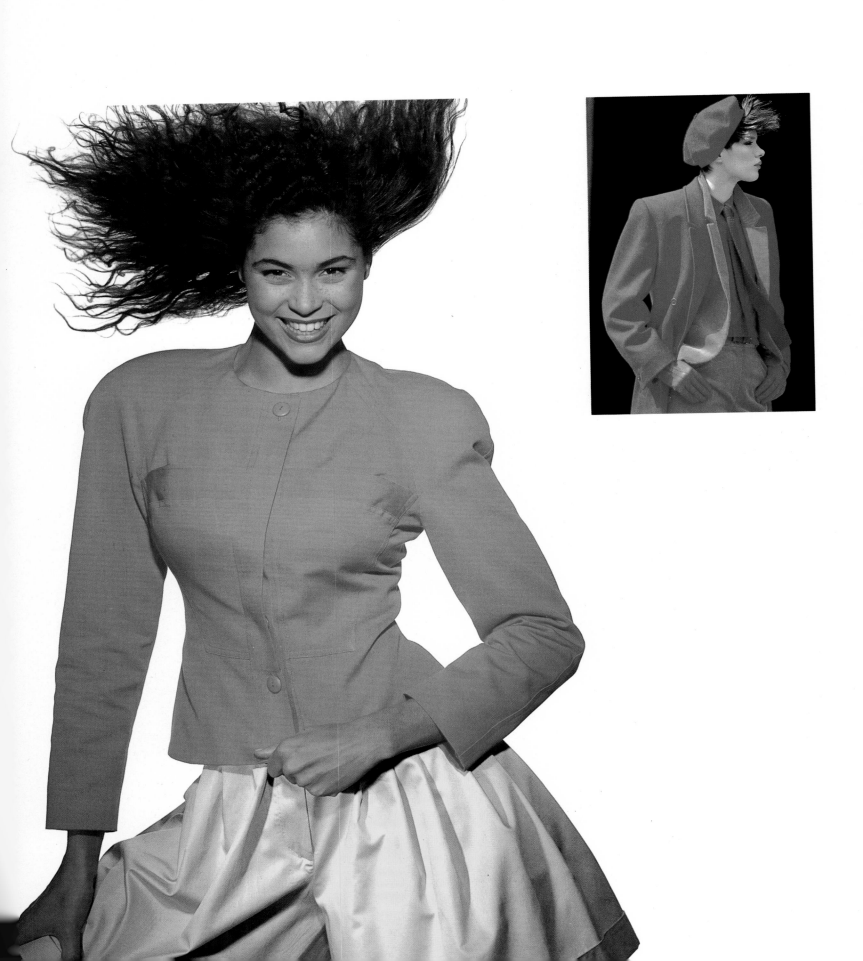

ACCENT ON COLOUR

Use bold shades, individually or in striking combinations to punctuate your appearance!

Bright, fun colours should not simply be reserved for summer days or parties. Go for bold whatever the season, whatever the occasion and enjoy the impact of vibrant colour. Strong colours are also mood boosters – who could feel down wearing sunshine yellow? Some shades are linked with certain emotions – red spells passion, for example, blue calmness and tranquility, while purple has spiritual associations. Put them together and you have an explosive mixture!

Left, main picture Eye-catching colours in simple lines – an orange, fitted jacket is great with loose, full-cut lime shorts.
Left, inset Clashing colours can work together; the red and orange layers look fun. Other unexpected but successful mixtures are purple and orange,

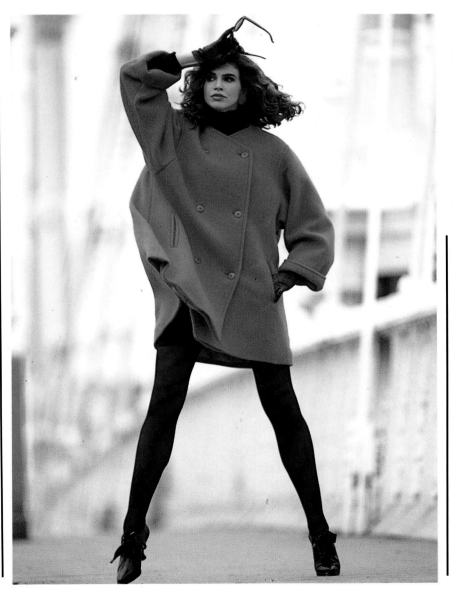

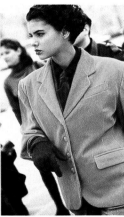

red and green, and yellow and pink.
Above Rich textures and colours are combined: a fine corduroy, tailored mustard jacket is dressed up with subtle, deep shades of red in the velvet tie and blue for the gloves.
Left A colourful coat will chase away winter blues! Short and beautifully cut, this coat would look great over tapered trousers. Here, the mauve is complemented by black accessories, but a vibrant scarf could be added as well.

SPOT ON

Switch on to spots, dots, checks and stripes. These graphic patterns can make the most casual outfit look super sharp.

You want to look smart for a special occasion – but not overdressed. What's the answer? Choose easy shapes in spots, checks and stripes. These high-powered patterns sharpen up every item of clothing, from pyjama pants to long, pleated skirts; from classic, loose-cut T-shirts to fitted tops and jackets.

These are some of the most adaptable clothes you can buy. You can team a sporty, striped T-shirt with summery shorts one day, and wear the same top with city slick trousers and a blazer jacket the next.

Mixing different sizes of stripes, spots and checks together looks snappy: put a big, narrow-stripe shirt over broad-stripe trousers, or a microdot blouse with a bold coin-spot skirt.

You can optimize on optical effects by wearing stripes with

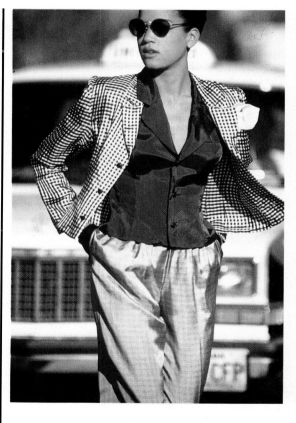

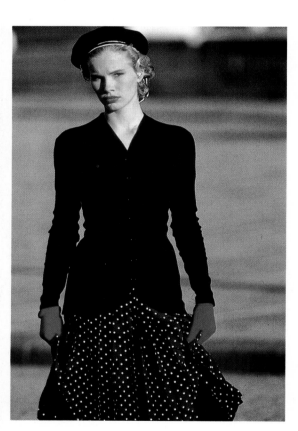

spots and stripes with checks, when the fabrics are of similar textures and the colourway of the two garments is the same. Use spotted, checked or striped accessories to give an extra lift to plain outfits too.

The freshest effects usually come with contrasts of black or dark navy with white, or bold primary colours, but for a complete change of mood, try spotted pastel colours in soft, elegant fabrics.

Above, left Playing with patterns – a silk checker-board fitted jacket can be worn over a plain shirt or on its own. Teamed with silky Prince of Wales check trousers, this combination is terrific for after-work dates.

Above Easy-to-wear elegance from a classic polka dot pleated cotton skirt worn with a body-sculpting black cotton jacket. The red gloves and jaunty beret give this outfit an extra special touch.

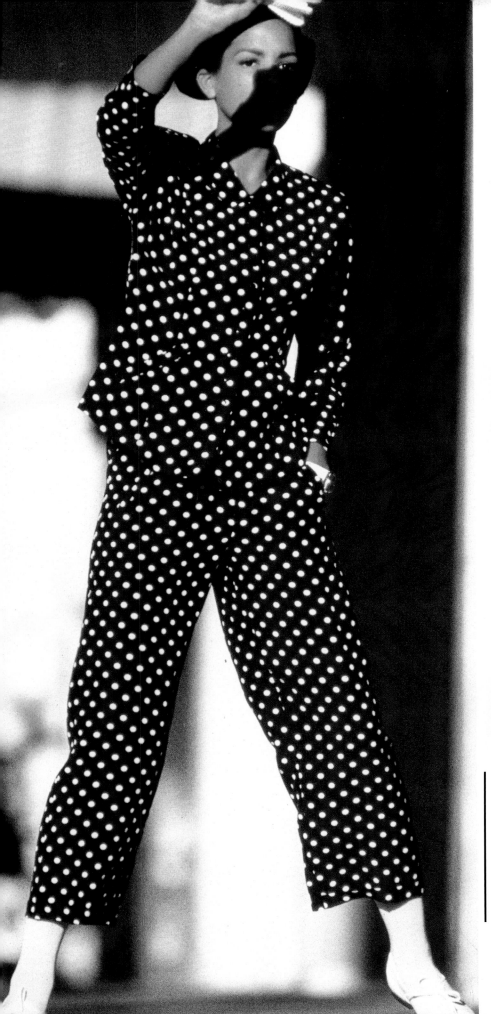

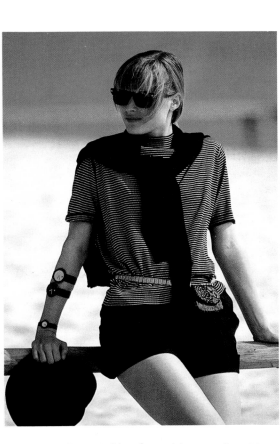

Right The elegant side of sporty – a boldly-printed, coin-spot two-piece sets the pace. White gloves, fine cotton socks and white leather brogues complete the look. You could wear the cropped trousers with a white or red vest top for sunny weekends and wear the shirt with a short and tight, or long, pleated skirt. *Above* The casual look of a narrow-stripe T-shirt is matched with black shorts and sweater and a soft hat.

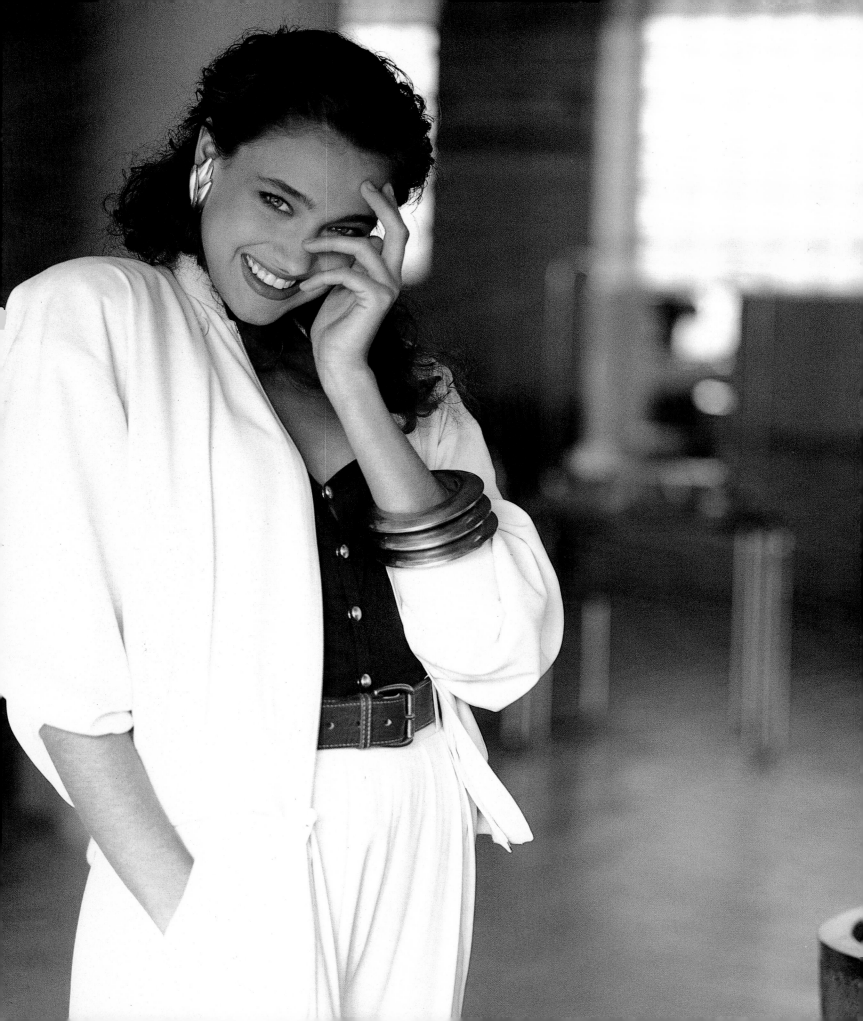

SUMMER IN THE CITY

Here's how to look polished and keep your cool when the heat is on!

Rising temperatures don't mean you have to lose your sense of style. Even in the city, cool clothes can still be stunningly smart. Clever buys are a pair of bermuda shorts and a well-cut, lightweight jacket. The only white shoes worth having are flat canvas or leather pumps (leather is permeable, allowing feet to breathe) or low-heeled strappy sandals. High white shoes rarely look good. White is a great colour choice for clothes as it looks clean and fresh and will emphasize a glowing tan. Chunky metallic accessories complement a warmer skin tone for day or the evening. Brightly coloured glass beads are fabulous for a more casual, fun image.

Main picture Cool and comfortable to wear, yet elegant, a cream trouser suit is worn with a fitted, button-through navy bodice. Bold gold jewellery and a brown belt give the outfit extra style.
Right A collarless shaped jacket in crisp whiter-than-white looks expensive because of its cut and detailing. Add a lace body.

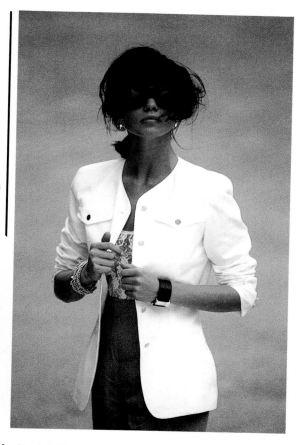

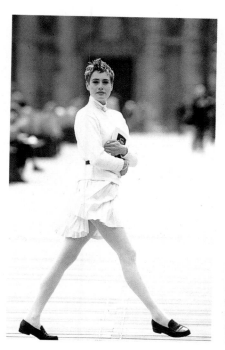

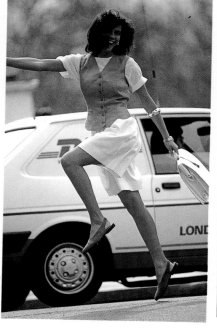

Far left Even if the sun disappears behind a cloud, white can still look right. This creamy white cotton knit jumper and short pleated skirt with opaque tights will keep the wearer warm.

Left Cutting a dash in tailored bermuda shorts: the waistcoat adds interest to an otherwise basic outfit of shorts and T-shirt. Silver jewellery — bangles and ear-rings — dresses it up.

MAKING HEADLINES

Hats are big fashion news. After many years in the style doldrums, they have made an important revival in womenswear.

A hat is the ultimate short cut to style. They are being worn casually and formally, stamping the wearer's personality on to the clothes.

Hats for formal occasions carry larger price tags than casual hats and are often works of art, exquisitely shaped and finely detailed.

When trying on a hat, use a full-length mirror so that you can consider the whole silhouette. Remember that you can change the trims – add veils, bows, rosettes – to suit different occasions. If you want to give a natural straw hat a fresh look, spray it with glossy paint.

Men's hatters are a good source of well-made panamas and modern felt bowlers. Invest in cardboard hat boxes – you could cover them in striped paper, for instance, and make them a feature of a room.

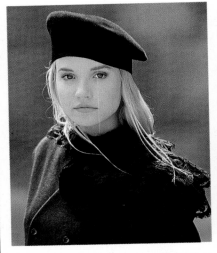
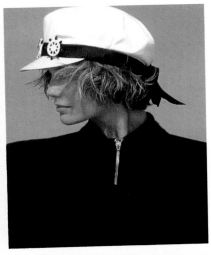
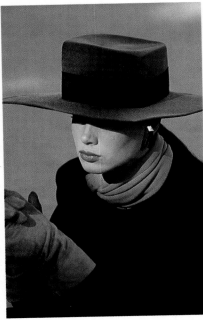
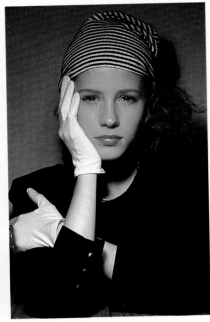

Left top A crisp, peaked sailor-style hat is worn low over the forehead and decorated with nautical badges.

Far left, A traditional beret on a broad band looks strong and stylish in black. It is worn plain here with a fancy lace-collared top and tailored jacket. Add brooches to make it casual and street-trendy.

Far left, below Deep-crowned with a striking wide brim, this dramatic hat makes a super-confident statement.

Left, below A striped, soft cotton pull-on hat is perfect for cooler weather. Worn with pristine white gloves, a very casual hat looks elegant and chic.

Right A stunning straw boater with an extra-large brim has a black band which makes it look contemporary and sharp. Large, bold silver ear-rings balance the look.

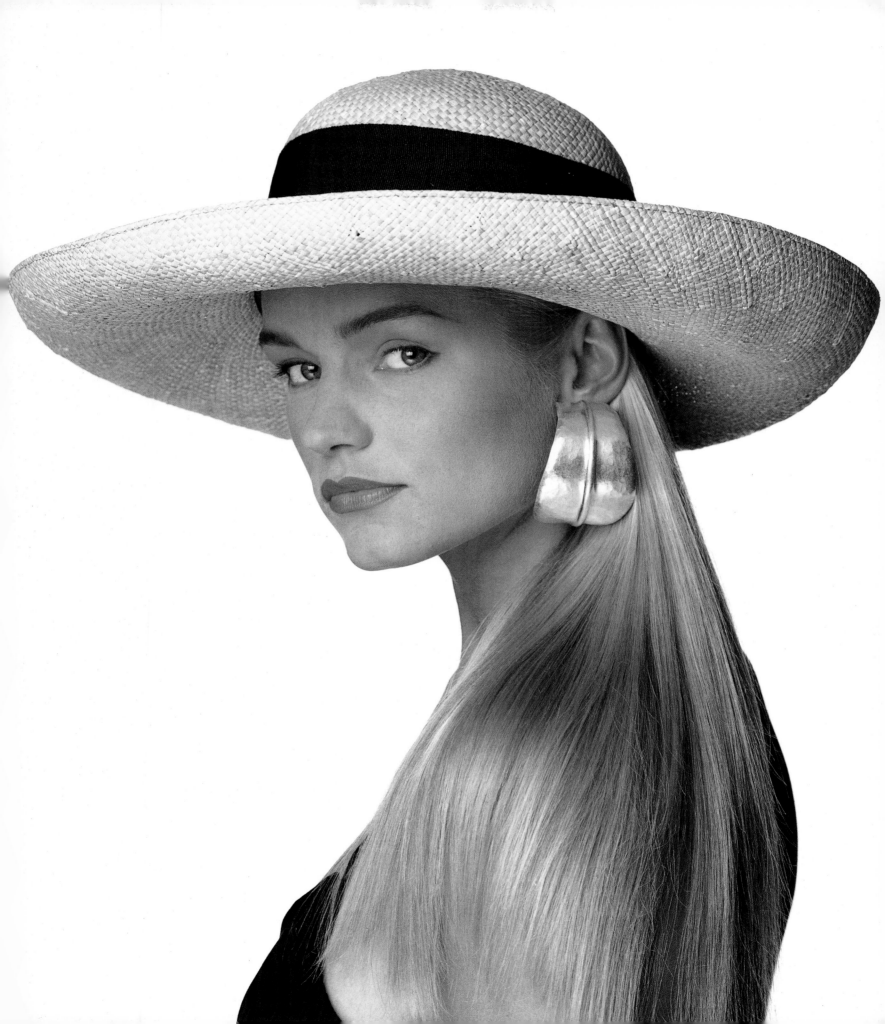

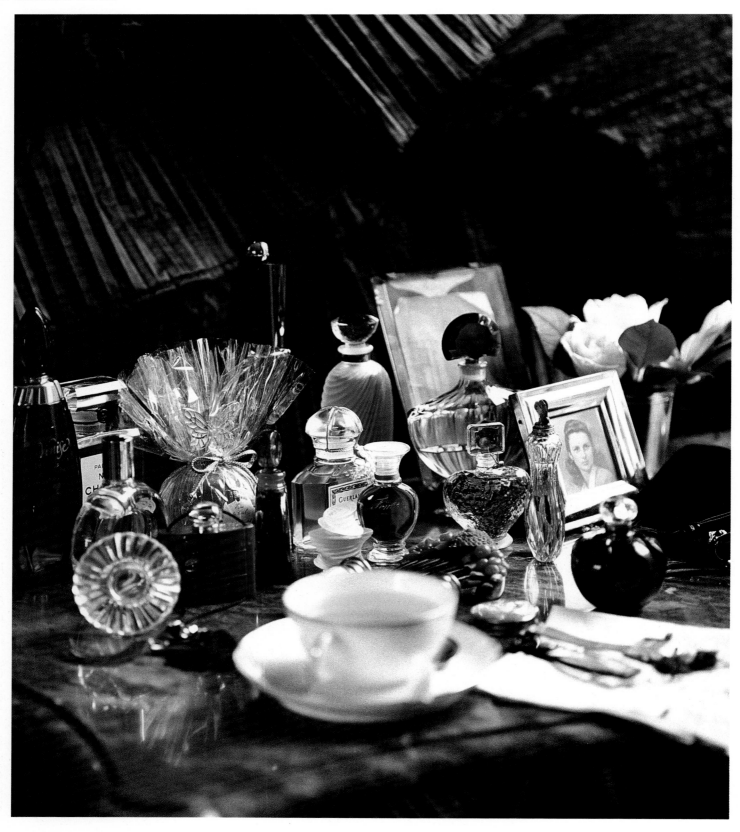

FRAGRANCE NOTES

Scent can be sensuous or romantic,
a fashion statement or a reflection of your personality.

Fragrance is as much part of your image as the clothes you wear. While the notion of one 'signature' fragrance that you wore every day used to be popular, the trend now is to have a 'wardrobe' of fragrances – a selection of scents to wear on different occasions, at different times of the day or year.

Fragrance is an instant pick-you-up: it can match or brighten your mood, influence other people's impression of you and bring back memories.

A psychologist, Joachim Mensing, pioneered the link between fragrance and personality types and developed a test to identify who chooses which scent. Extrovert, optimistic types, for instance, tend to choose fresh, floral fragrances, while oriental, spicy scents with a floral hint can suit more introverted personalities who enjoy a relatively ordered, uncomplicated life.

THE RIGHT FRAGRANCE
● Don't buy a fragrance just because it smells good on someone you know. Scents react differently to individual skin chemistry. Test it on yourself before buying.
● Testing a fragrance by sniffing it from the bottle only gives an impression of the top note, which soon evaporates; the middle or 'body' of a fragrance interacts with your skin and the base note is the foundation of the fragrance, the longest lasting part of the 'harmony' or blend of ingredients. Apply some to your wrist and walk around for a while, letting it 'dry down', observing how it changes on you.
● Don't test more than a small number of fragrances at a time or your nose will become confused. Leave as much time as possible between testing each one.
● Eau de cologne is the weakest form of fragrance, followed by eau de toilette. Eau de parfum and esprit de parfum are stronger, with parfum, or perfume, being the most concentrated and therefore longest lasting. As a general rule, go for subtle eau de cologne and eau de toilette during the day. The stronger concentrates work better in the evening.
● Think about the climate in which your new fragrance will be worn. Warm, humid atmospheres intensify most scents, whereas dry heat weakens them. In some cases, cool, damp weather brings out their true character.

Fragrance for effect
Apply fragrance to pulse points on the body – on your wrists, around your neck, the backs of your knees. Spray a little on freshly washed hair.

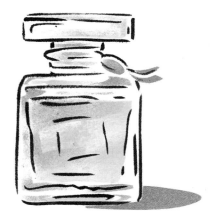

Layering fragrance ensures that it's kept subtle, yet gives a lasting effect. Start with a scented shower gel or body lotion in the morning. Later in the day, revive the scent with a spritz of eau de toilette, and add perfume in the evening.

Keeping fragrance fresh
Keep your fragrance in its box, away from bright sunlight and extremes of heat or cold to avoid unnecessary deterioration. Ensure the stopper is tight on the bottle to prevent evaporation.

Once opened, a scent will last six months to a year, stored correctly. Don't save it just for special occasions over the years, as it will no longer be in peak condition.

MAXIMIZING YOUR PERFUME
Once you've finished your perfume, leave the bottle without the cap in your underwear drawer or at the bottom of your wardrobe to scent your clothes subtly.

INDEX

ACKNOWLEDGMENTS

The publisher thanks the following photographers and organizations for their permission to reproduce the photographs in this book:

12 Transworld Features; 16 Camera Press; 17 Transworld Features; 18 Robert Erdmann/Cosmopolitan Magazine; 19 Rapho/Donnezan; 20 left Transworld Features; 20 right Camera Press; 21 left Transworld Features; 22 above Transworld Features; 22 centre Kelly/The Image Bank; 22 below Longfield/The Image Bank; 23 above Steve E. Landis/Cosmopolitan Magazine; 23 below Rapho/Donnezan; 24 left Transworld Features; 24 above right Transworld Features; 24 below right Visalli/The Image Bank; 33 Costantino Ruspoli/Cosmopolitan Magazine; 34–5 Marie Claire/Chatelain; 42–43 Cent Idees/G. Chabaneix/G. Chabaneix; 44–5 Sandra Lousada/Cosmopolitan Magazine; 46 Transworld Features; 47 above Transworld Features; 47 below left Camera Press; 47 below right Marie Claire/Chatelain; 49 Camera Press; 51 Camera Press; 52 Transworld Features; 53 Transworld Features; 54 Camera Press; 55 above Camera Press; 55 below Transworld Features; 57 above Bucourt/Box Office; 57 below Nabon/Box Office; 59 Transworld Features; 60 Marie Claire Bis/L'Harmeroult; 61 Camera Press; 62–3 Transworld Features; 64 Transworld Features; 65 Lutz/Box Office; 66–7 Transworld Features; 70 Tom Wool/Cosmopolitan Magazine; 81 Tim Bret-Day/Cosmopolitan Magazine; 83 right Robert Erdmann/Cosmopolitan Magazine; 83 left Costantino Ruspoli/Cosmopolitan Magazine; 84 Camera Press; 86 Tim Bret-Day/Cosmopolitan Magazine; 87 right Nicola Ranaldi/Cosmopolitan Magazine; 88 Marie Claire/Sacha; 90 Camera Press; 93 Christof Gstalder/Cosmopolitan Magazine; 96 Transworld Features; 99 Barto/The Image Bank; 100 Camera Press; 101 Costantino Ruspoli/Cosmopolitan Magazine; 102 Syndication International; 103 Boussard/Box Office; 105 left Explorer; 105 centre Camera Press; 105 right Marie Claire/Jouanneau; 106 Paul Alexander/Cosmopolitan Magazine; 107 left Steven E. Landis/Cosmopolitan Magazine; 107 above right Marie Claire/Ferri; 107 below right Camera Press; 108 Marie Claire/Jouanneau; 109 Hair by Vidal Sassoon; 110 Nabon/Box Office; 111 left Boussard/Box Office; 111 right Lutz/Box Office; 112 L'Oreal – Studio Line; 113 Hair by Vidal Sassoon; 115 above left Camera Press; 115 below left Robert Erdmann/Cosmopolitan Magazine; 116 left Costantino Ruspoli/Cosmopolitan Magazine; 116 centre Lutz/Box Office; 116 right Marie Claire/Moser; 117 Marie Claire/Sacha; 118 Boussard/Box Office; 119 above Costantino Ruspoli/Cosmopolitan Magazine; 119 centre Lutz/Box Office; 119 below Camera Press; 120–1 Transworld Features; 122–4 Costantino Ruspoli/Cosmopolitan Magazine; 127–9 Transworld Features; 132 Costantino Ruspoli/Cosmopolitan Magazine; 136 Transworld Features; 138 Sean Knox/Cosmopolitan Magazine; 139–40 Camera Press; 141 Robert Erdmann/Cosmopolitan Magazine; 143 Transworld Features; 144 Tim Bret-Day/Cosmopolitan Magazine; 146 Chris Craymer/Cosmopolitan Magazine; 147–9 Transworld Features; 149 left Marie Claire/Bucourt; 149 right Transworld Features; 150 Tim Bret-Day/Cosmopolitan Magazine; 151 above left Sean Knox/Cosmopolitan Magazine; 151 below left Transworld Features; 151 above right Marie Claire/Sacha; 151 below right Natalie Lamoral/Cosmopolitan Magazine; 152 left Transworld Features; 152 centre Nick Briggs/Cosmopolitan Magazine; 152 right Marie Claire/Bucourt; 153 Natalie Lamoral/Cosmopolitan Magazine; 154 above Marie Claire/Carrera; 154 below Transworld Features; 155 Transworld Features; 156 left Camera Press; 156 right Chris Craymer/Cosmopolitan Magazine; 157 left Chris Craymer/Cosmopolitan Magazine;; 157 right Transworld Features; 158 left Tim Bret-Day/Cosmopolitan Magazine; 158 right Cent Idees/Jacobs; 159 left Marie Claire/Bucourt; 159 above right Marie Claire/Sacha; 159 below right Brynner/Box Office; 160 Eammon McCabe/Cosmopolitan Magazine; 161 left Eammon McCabe/Cosmopolitan Magazine; 161 right Transworld Features; 162 left Sean Knox/Cosmopolitan Magazine; 162 centre Marie Claire/Moser; 162 right Graham Peebles/Cosmopolitan Magazine; 163 Tony McGee/Cosmopolitan Magazine; 164 left Tony McGee/Cosmopolitan Magazine;; 164 right Marie Claire/Sacha; 165 left Natalie Lamoral/Cosmopolitan Magazine; 165 right Marie Claire Bis/Schmidt; 166 left Marie Claire/Kohli; 166 right Marie Claire/Carrera; 167 left Marie Claire/Kohli; 167 right Transworld Features; 168 Nicola Ranaldi/Cosmopolitan Magazine; 169 left Marie Claire/Carrera; 169 centre and right Tim Bret-Day/Cosmopolitan Magazine; 170 above left Transworld Features; 170 below left Marie Claire/Moser; 170 above right Transworld Features; 170 below right Marie Claire/Hiett; 171 Syndication International; 172 Cent Idees/N.de Noussac/I.Garcon.

Special photography by Anthony Crickmay and Iain Philpott for Conran Octopus:
Anthony Crickmay 1, 3, 4–5, 8, 10, 21 right, 26, 27, 28, 29, 30, 31, 32, 35 above, 36, 37, 38, 39. Iain Philpott 40, 41, 72, 74, 75, 77, 78–9, 80, 92, 94.

Make-up and hair pages 1, 3, 4–5, 8, 10, 21 right, 26, 27, 28, 29, 30, 32, 35 above, 36, 37, 38, 39 by Teresa Fairminer.
Pages 40, 41, 72, 74, 75, 77, 78, 79, 80, 92, 94: make-up by Jenny Nolan; hair by Derek Thompson of Michaeljohn.

Author's Acknowledgments
The authors wish to thank Hilary Arnold, Cortina Butler, Karen Bowen, Jessica Walton and Rosanna Kelly of Conran Octopus; Pamela Todd of A.P. Watt; Emma Dally, Deny Filmer, Joan Tinney and Lisa Podmore of Cosmopolitan; Esme Newton-Dunn; Clayton Marshall; Russ Malkin; Anthony Crickmay; Iain Philpott; John Prothero and Derek Thompson of Michaeljohn; Teresa Fairminer; Jenny Nolan; Caroline Eversfield and Stephen Glass of Face Facts; Dance Bizarre; Jesse James; The Conran Shop; Graham Smith at Kangol.